D0093796

BLAST THE SUGAR OUT!

ALSO BY IAN K. SMITH, M.D.

BLAST THE SUGAR OUT!

Lower Blood Sugar, Lose Weight, Live Better

Ian K. Smith, M.D.

St. Martin's Press ≈ New York

BLAST THE SUGAR OUT! Copyright © 2017 by Ian K. Smith. All rights reserved. Printed in the United States of America. For information, address St. Martin's Press, 175 Fifth Avenue, New York, N.Y. 10010.

www.stmartins.com

The Library of Congress Cataloging-in-Publication Data is available upon request.

ISBN 978-1-250-13013-6 (hardcover)
ISBN 978-1-250-13014-3 (e-book)

Our books may be purchased in bulk for promotional, educational, or business use. Please contact your local bookseller or the Macmillan Corporate and Premium Sales Department at 1-800-221-7945, extension 5442, or by e-mail at MacmillanSpecialMarkets@macmillan.com.

First Edition: April 2017

10 9 8 7 6 5 4 3 2 1

To my twin brother, Dana. Friend. Confidant. Road Dog. Fellow Warrior. You've always made the ride interesting at the peaks and in the valleys. The 5 A.M. preschool hill runs will forever mold my strength. Eternally bonded to you and in love.

CONTENTS

INTRODUCTION

When I was just a young first-year medical student, my grandmother, the anchor of our family, was diagnosed with type 2 diabetes. This was a tremendously difficult blow to her, and thus the entire family, because she had been healthy all of her life and never required medications or therapeutic interventions. She was scared, and so were the rest of us as we struggled to understand not just why she was so unlucky, but what could be done to make sure that she avoided all of the devastating complications that can come from the disease.

Everyone looked to me because I was supposed to be the medical expert in the family. But the truth was that I knew virtually nothing about diabetes; I was just in my first semester of my first year. My reaction was like it always had been when facing a challenge—take it head-on without fear and work extremely hard to conquer it. So I searched for and digested every particle of information about diabetes and what could be done to make a difference. The more I researched and learned, the more convinced I became that diabetes was not a death sentence like so many of us think. It was controllable through lifestyle behaviors, as well as appropriate medicinal therapy if necessary.

I went home for the holiday that winter, sat my grandmother down, and explained to her as best as I could what I had learned and what I thought would make her life as normal as possible. She listened and she cried, not because she was scared, but because I had given her back the hope that had vanished the second her doctor had announced her diagnosis. The first thing we did was change her eating habits. An old woman from the South, her typical cuisine was loaded with fried foods and sugary treats. Sugar and butter have long been the centerpiece of Southern cuisine and thus the foundation of many of the foods that we ate at home. We immediately cut back on not just how many carbohydrates she consumed but the types of carbohydrates. Getting them from better sources was important in controlling her blood sugar, and this was a change that could be made immediately.

The second thing we did was go down to the local gym, where she signed up for a membership. This doesn't sound too groundbreaking now, but my grandmother was a plump little church lady who probably hadn't exercised regularly in fifty years. At the time I took her to the gym, it was not common to see senior citizens there exercising with the younger crowd with loud music piping in from the ceiling speakers. I had been an athlete all of my life, and although I was new to medicine, I was a veteran sportsman. My brother and I taught her the machines and devised a little workout for her that was challenging enough but also something she could actually do. Here she was, my little grandmother in pants and sneakers, walking her hardest on that treadmill next to a 250-pound football player trying to do wind sprints. It's an image that I will never forget.

After three weeks of better eating (not perfect, but better) and a regimen of exercise (four days a week, about 20 to 35 minutes each time), my grandmother went back to the doctor for a follow-up visit. I will never forget what she said when I talked to her on the phone from school. The first thing the doctor said when he got the results of her blood work was, "What have you been doing? Your blood sugar levels have gone down so much." My grandmother proudly told him that she was watching her sweets and that she was exercising. The next thing he told her brought tears to our eyes. "I am going to have to cut your medication in half, because your sugars are so low you don't need that much anymore."

Diabetes can be frustrating and challenging and exhausting, but for the vast majority of people who live with it, it is manageable and controllable. My grandmother did it without many of the resources or facts that are known today. She, too, was scared and sad, facing changes in her senior years that were revolutionary and unthinkable. But she executed simple lifestyle changes that made a big difference in her life, and she no longer felt like her diabetes was controlling her; she was controlling it. Eighty million people are thought to be prediabetic—on the verge of true diabetes—and most don't even know how close they are to that precipice.

This book is designed not only for prediabetics and those with diabetes but also for anyone who simply wants to cut down on sugar consumption, lose weight, and lead the healthiest life possible. In just five weeks, you can take your life back and regain control of your health destiny, avoiding a lifetime of chronic and life-interrupting illness. Blast the Sugar Out and put the life back in!

—*Ian K. Smith, M.D.*
April 2017

BLAST THE SUGAR OUT!

1 HOW *BLAST THE SUGAR OUT* WORKS

My brother, Dana, without my knowing, decided that he was going to drastically reduce sugar in his diet. He felt like he had been eating too many sweets—powdered donuts, candy bars, and sweetened drinks. A supreme athlete his entire life, he felt like his body was not responding like it always had and his energy levels were down. He had an overall feeling of discomfort and wasn't sure what was causing it.

After an exhausting day, he sat down on his couch and thought about his diet and exercise plan. He is a marathon runner and runs several miles a day as easy as the average person walks up a flight of stairs. The exercise wasn't his problem. So, he took a closer look at his eating and started realizing that he was snacking out of convenience or as a result of urges, and grabbing sweets around the clock. A candy bar between meetings, donuts late at night on the way home from work, his day was literally covered in sugar.

The next day he used the same determination that had powered him through many successes throughout his life to eliminate the added sugars from his diet and quit cold turkey all bingeing on sweets. He later explained to me that it was not exactly easy at first. His body was so accustomed to its daily sugar hits that when it no longer received them it let him know. Mild headaches, lagging energy levels, and stomach discomfort was all the evidence he needed that his body had become addicted to those hidden sugars. In just a couple of weeks, however, it all changed. The headaches and stomach discomfort went away and his energy levels soared. He told me that he felt brand-new—as if he had been given his life back. He ran stronger, wasn't feeling sluggish in the middle of the day, and even felt like his mind was sharper and more productive.

My brother recognized what so many health experts have been trying to convey for so long. Sugar is addictive and powerful and in excessive quantities can take a toll on your health. My brother had not reached the stage where he was diagnosed with any medical condition, but a steady march of weeks and months and years of sugar overindulgence will surely take their toll even on the most chiseled and athletic body. Imagine what it can do to those who are not so athletically inclined and who don't have anything to offset its impact.

The simple truth is that many are not as fortunate as my brother and have been diagnosed with prediabetes or type 2 diabetes. But it's important to emphasize that these diagnoses are not a death sentence; they are a wake-up call. Your body is telling you that you need to eat differently, exercise better, and make smarter lifestyle choices. Those who have been diagnosed with diabetes are not alone in this fight by any stretch of the imagination. In the United States, an estimated 29.1 million people have diabetes, and 8.1 million of them are walking around with the disease and don't even know they have it. Every year, an astounding 1.4 million Americans are newly diagnosed with the dreaded statement, "You have diabetes." But as enormous as those statistics are, there's one that's even bigger. Eighty-six million Americans aged twenty years and older have prediabetes, which means they're on the fence. If they don't change the way they eat and become more physically active, they will develop the full-blown disease and carry the diagnosis. What should be extremely concerning to everyone is that these numbers over the last ten years have gotten worse, not better. And if the physical and mental costs that come along with the disease are not enough, the financial cost is also staggering—$245 billion dollars a year, with $176 billion due to direct medical costs and $69 billion due to reduced productivity in the workplace.

Blast the Sugar Out! is specifically designed to help those who are prediabetic, diabetic, or anyone who simply wants to reduce sugar consumption and lose weight. This five-week plan has been built with three major tenets in place: simple, affordable, and effective. Millions of people have followed and lost tremendous amounts of weight on my *SHRED Diet* series (*SHRED*, *SUPER SHRED*, and *SHRED Power Cleanse*). Many of them were diabetics who took those programs and modified them to make them fit what they needed to do within the restrictions of their condition. Not only did they lose weight, but they lowered their blood sugar levels and their need for medications and felt so much better. Well, *Blast the Sugar Out!* is a plan that is built specifically for those who have been warned that they are prediabetic and need to make changes, as well as those who have been diagnosed with the full-blown disease. Diabetes is preventable and controllable, and over these next five weeks you will learn how to *shred* the disease!

Each week is composed of daily meal plans that are straightforward and laid out in a way that gives you flexibility. You will be given choices throughout the day to accommodate food/drink preferences as well as convenience factors, such as what you have readily available to eat and what is most affordable on your budget. No two diabetics are alike, and you know your body and disease better than anyone. So if you need to avoid certain foods that are on the plan, you should do that. If you need to modify the quantities or preparation of the menu items, you should do that as well. You know your triggers, so take those into consideration as you follow the plan.

HABITS

Each week starts out by helping you focus. All of us have good habits, bad habits, and habits that we can improve. Each week we are going to work on the 1–1–1 process. Break one bad habit; add one good habit; and improve one habit. It's important that you not just think about these three habits, but that you actually write them down on day 1 at the beginning of each week. By the time you have completed the five weeks, you should have broken five bad habits, added five good habits, and improved five habits.

Here is an example of what it might look like:

WEEK 1, DAY 1

BAD HABIT: Eating too much fast food.
CHANGE: Reduce the weekly number of fast food meals in half.
GOOD HABIT: Not skipping breakfast even if I'm running late.
IMPROVED HABIT: Exercising.
CHANGE: Exercise 4 times a week instead of the 2 times a week that I currently do.

SCHEDULE

When it comes to controlling diabetes, it's not just what you eat and how much, but when you eat, that can make a big difference. Consistency in your meal timing can be extremely important in keeping your blood-sugar levels stable. Although it might not be possible to eat at the same time every day, consuming your meals within 30 to 45 minutes of a regularly scheduled time can make a difference.

Create a schedule that works for you. A simple guide that you might try to use is to eat your breakfast at least within an hour of getting up. Try to position your snacks directly between your meals. If you have breakfast at 8 A.M. and lunch at 12 P.M., try to have your snack at 10 A.M. Your dinner might be at 7 P.M., so the snack between lunch and dinner should be around 3:30 P.M. If your day calls for a third snack, you can have that at any time after 90 minutes past your dinner. In the example below, the snack would be 8:30 P.M. or later. Please note that not all days call for a post-dinner snack, so make sure you pay attention to each day's plan.

The example below is just one possible schedule, but you should adjust your timing based on when you wake up in the morning and set the rest of the day from there.

Awake	Breakfast	Snack	Lunch	Snack	Dinner	Snack
7 A.M.	8 A.M.	10 A.M.	12 P.M.	3:30 P.M.	7 P.M.	8:30 P.M.

Try to stick to your schedule as closely as possible, and do your best to avoid skipping meals. Your body will grow accustomed to eating at certain times, but consuming your meals and snacks irregularly will get in the way of you regulating hormones, sugar levels, and your metabolism. Please note that in week 4 you will have a very different schedule than in the other four weeks. A sample time schedule is included in that week's chapter.

MAIN DISH CHOICES

You have choices for your main dish. If none of the choices are available to you, please try to make a substitution that is as close as possible to the choices. If you have an allergy or a dietary preference such as vegetarian or vegan, you can make the appropriate substitutions. Salads and vegetables are always acceptable as a substitution for a meal. For example, if the meal plan calls for a chicken sandwich or turkey wrap, you can opt for a salad or three servings of vegetables. You can also opt for one or two cups of soup.

POWER UPS

The Power Ups are like side dishes. They are part of your meal. You can have them if you'd like or not have them. You can eat part of the serving or all of it. Eat until your satiated, but don't eat until your stuffed.

SNACKS

Snacks can be extremely helpful when losing weight. They can help prevent you from overeating during mealtime, which is important because overindulging at one sitting can disrupt hormone levels as well as destabilize blood-sugar levels. Each day has snacks built into the program. These snacks are optional but highly recommended. Chapter 8 has more than 100 snack options that you can choose from. These snacks are broken down into how many carbohydrates they contain. If you prefer to eat a snack that is not on the list, you are free to do so, but you must follow the carbohydrate guidelines of the recommended snack. If the snack during a given day calls for 10 grams or less of carbohydrates, make sure you look at the total carbs number in the nutritional label of your substitute.

It is important that you consult your health-care team to make sure you are still following the guidelines and suggestions that were made. You should team up with your health-care provider; as a team, you know and understand your diabetes best. Diabetics respond differently to therapy and nutrition. How your blood sugar levels fluctuate can be completely different from someone else who takes the same medication or eats the same food or does the same exercise. It's important to monitor your blood sugar levels while on the plan and make adjustments if necessary.

This book is a well-researched, scientifically-based guide, but not the final word on what you should and shouldn't do. Pay attention to your body and the way it responds, and that will help you make smart decisions.

BEVERAGES

It's important to make smart beverage choices. Your goal should be to drink plenty of **water** each day—as much as 6–8 cups. You should avoid sugary drinks that have little, if any, nutritional value. **Sodas** are a prime example of what you want to limit or avoid altogether, even if it's diet soda. **Fruit-infused water** is always a great option if plain water is simply too bland for you. You can also try **sparkling water**, as the fizz is often more satisfying to many. When shopping for canned or bottled drinks, please be careful of the carbohydrate and sugar content. Our aim is to reduce the amount of unnecessary carbs and unfortunately, many beverages have lots of hidden sugars that you don't need and should avoid. **Fruit juices** have sugar in them. However, they are natural sugars and they are part of a larger package that is healthier than soda. Fruit juices contain vitamins, fiber, and other important phytonutrients, but make sure you are drinking 100 percent juice. **Fresh juice** is always best and you should choose those fruit juices that are clearly marked "No Sugar Added." Depending on your blood sugar levels, you should monitor how much fruit juice you consume as even the natural sugars can cause a spike in your levels. However, if the option is soda versus fruit juice, the choice is very clear—fruit juice. **Coffee** is allowed. One cup per day, as clean as possible. A little sugar and milk/cream is allowed, but very small amounts. **Teas** are allowed, but opt for unsweetened teas. If you drink **alcohol**, try to limit the amount you consume to no more than 1 drink per day. One drink for the purposes of this program would be 1 glass of wine or one bottle of beer or one mixed drink. Please don't overdo it as alcohol can contain lots of sugars and calories.

EXERCISE

This is a critical component to any successful weight loss strategy, and it is a critical one for anyone trying to lower their blood-sugar levels or reduce the effects of excess sugar on their body. You can decrease your percentage of body fat, increase the effectiveness of your insulin, and prevent wild swings in your blood sugar levels by following the exercise plan in this book. Each day provides the amount and type of exercise that you should do. Some days, there will be just a cardiovascular/aerobic suggestion, and other days there will be resistance training added. There will be some days when you have a rest day. The exercise times provided are minimal suggestions. By all means, if you want to exercise more, go ahead and do it safely. The appendices, pages 209–212, contain suggestions for the types of exercises that fit the categories of cardiovascular/aerobic and resistance training.

Choose exercises that fit your lifestyle and that are fun and challenge you without being too difficult to accomplish. Try a variety of exercises. Doing the same thing all the time not only can get a little boring, but it can lose its effectiveness over time as the body becomes accustomed to the same type of exercise. If for some reason you miss your exercise on a day that has it listed, no problem. Do that exercise the next day and move the other days accordingly.

Rest days don't mean sit on your couch and do nothing. These are days when you allow your body to recover because your body needs time to heal and rebuild even after small amounts of exercise. A rest day still means that you can go for a nice walk and get your heart rate going and your muscles contracting. It's just not as intense and concentrated of an exercise session as you would typically have during one of the active exercise days.

MAINTENANCE

The major goal of the five-week plan is that you develop a lifestyle that includes making wise nutritional choices along with establishing a regular, enjoyable regimen of exercise. After the five weeks, if you have not hit your weight goal, feel free to do another cycle, but this time switch the order of the weeks that you follow. If you are happy with your weight, simply continue to eat and exercise the way you now know how to do without necessarily following the program strictly as written. This is about you learning how to live the rest of your life so that you can prevent the onset of diabetes, or if you already have it, so that you can control it and not be constantly burdened.

If you decide not to do a second cycle right away after completing the first, that is not a problem. But what you shouldn't do is return to eating how you were in the past and not exercising effectively. This will only bring the weight back and cause havoc on your blood sugar levels. You have worked so hard to make progress; don't just throw it all away.

Remember, this is not about making quick changes that you won't stick with. This is all about making lifestyle changes that are going to keep you healthy and active for the rest of your life. Once completing a cycle or two of the program, you don't need to follow the book verbatim. I want you to be able to make smart decisions based on your new knowledge and what you've learned over the last several weeks. But just as a car needs to go to the repair shop periodically for tune-ups to check the tires and brakes and change the oil, the same is true when it comes to our bodies and how we nourish and move them. It's easy to get a little off track—all of us do. But when you find this has happened, don't get discouraged and down on yourself. Instead, pick one or two weeks of the plan and follow those weeks as a tune-up. This book is now your trusted companion; you should refer to it in times of need or doubt or when you simply need a little reassurance!

2 THE SKINNY ON SUGAR

Sugar is everywhere. Cookies, cakes, soda, fruit, salads, cereal, juice—it's almost impossible not to sit down to a meal and not have some amount of sugar on your plate. The United States, like many other countries, has become a sugar nation. Our consumption is the highest that it's ever been, with some reports revealing that the average American consumes 156 pounds of sugars each year—the equivalent of thirty-one 5-pound bags. Sixty-six of those pounds come in the form of added sugars that carry with them no nutritional value. For a little perspective, the American Heart Association recommends that men consume no more than 36 grams of added sugar each day and that women consume no more than 24 grams. If you were to drink just one 20 oz can of soda, which has as much as 60 grams of sugar, you would be well over the recommendation and that's before taking your first bite of food.

What is sugar? Although to most it's the white granular crystals that we sprinkle on our cereal in the morning or pour in our coffee, it all starts with plants. Sugar is a type of carbohydrate. If you remember your old science lessons, plants make carbohydrates through a process called photosynthesis, where they take CO_2 (carbon dioxide) from the air, water from the ground, chlorophyll (green pigments that give plants their color), and sunlight. The results of photosynthesis are sucrose (sugar) and oxygen.

Sugar is naturally found in two plants—sugar beets and sugar cane. The process of obtaining sugar from these plants is fascinating.

SUGAR CONSUMPTION

American Heart Association recommends no more than 9.5 teaspoons per day

ACTUAL DAILY CONSUMPTION

AVERAGE ADULT:

22 Teaspoons per day

AVERAGE CHILD:

32 Teaspoons per day

Sugar in a bottle of cola

39 grams

Sugar in a bottle of snapple

36 grams

Sugar in a glazed donut

12 grams

Consumption: 156 pounds of sugar = thirty-one 5lb bags

The plant is washed, sliced, and soaked in hot water, which starts the process of separating the sugar from the rest of the plant. (In the case of sugar cane, the stalks are shredded before huge rollers crush the cane into a liquid mixture.) The result is a hot sugary liquid, which then gets filtered until what remains is a deep brown syrup. This deep brown color is due to the naturally occurring high molasses content of the plant. The deep brown syrup is allowed to slightly cool before being spun at high speed in a machine called a centrifuge—a basket with tiny holes in it that operates similar to a washing machine whirling during its spin cycle. During this phase, most of the molasses is spun away. The remaining light brown crystals are then sprayed with hot water to remove the remaining molasses and leave behind pure white sugar crystals. The sugar crystals are then dried. To develop the white granulated sugar that you use at your table, these crystals are decolorized so that there are no traces of the brown residue from the molasses. The last step is to run the crystals through filters so that impurities are removed and what remains are tiny, very fine crystals that you purchase at the store and pour into your sugar bowl.

The sugar that is obtained from sugar cane and sugar beets is the same sucrose that is found naturally in the original plants as well as fruits and vegetables. It's important to note that the body doesn't distinguish between the different types of sugar and thus breaks them down in exactly the same manner. The sucrose that you sprinkle onto your cereal is broken down the same way as the sucrose in your orange. However, whereas the sugar is the same and the body processes it the same way, you should know that the sugar in fruits and vegetables comes with powerful nutritional partners—antioxidants, fiber, vitamins, minerals, and other phytonutrients that are tremendously healthy. Although table sugar and fruit have the same type of sugar, remember that fruit comes with additional benefits, but table sugar or sugar in a can of soda has no nutritional value. If you're going to consume sugar—and we all do—think about the *sugar package* and focus on consuming those sugars that will provide a nutritional counterpunch.

Sucrose is what we typically refer to when we speak of sugar. When we consume sucrose, the body then breaks it down into individual sugar units of glucose and fructose. The body will typically use the glucose for energy, and the extra energy from fructose—if it's not needed—will be directed into the creation of that dreaded fat.

The other main sugars that are naturally found in food are glucose, fructose, lactose, and maltose. Glucose is the simple sugar that is the body's preferred energy source and circulates in our bloodstream. Most carbohydrates that we consume are broken down by the body into glucose. Fructose is a sugar that's naturally found in many fruits and vegetables. It's also added to various beverages such as fruit-flavored drinks, fruit juice cocktail drinks, and sodas. Fructose, however, is not the preferred energy source like glucose, for the brain or your muscles. It behaves differently in the body, potentially causing damage when its levels are too high and behaving more like fat in the body.

Lactose is a double sugar that contains a molecule of glucose and a molecule of galactose linked together. It's often called milk sugar because of where it's most commonly found. Lactose is the only common sugar of animal origin. Maltose also is a double sugar—two glucose molecules linked together. It's easily broken down by the body and often is used as a sweetening agent, as well as in food for infants who have a poor tolerance for lactose.

The following chart compares the different types of sugar in their relative sweetness to table sugar. Sucrose is assigned a sweetness value of 1; thus, those that are sweeter have a higher number and those that are not as sweet have a lower number.

SUGAR	RELATIVE SWEETNESS	COMMONLY KNOWN AS
Sucrose	1	Sugar
Glucose	0.7	Grape sugar
Fructose	1.1	Fruit sugar
Lactose	0.4	Milk sugar
Maltose	0.5	Malt sugar
Sorbitol	0.5	–

Source: *Asia Pacific Journal of Clinical Nutrition*

Sugar or carbohydrates are not just what we add to our food at the table. Many of our foods come loaded with sugar. Check out this chart from the University of Michigan's Comprehensive Diabetes Center. It lists some of the common foods/beverages that we consume and the amount of sugars/carbohydrates that they contain.

Bread Products	Portion Size	Carbs (g)
Bagel: Panera	1 plain bagel	60
Bread	1 regular slice	15–23
Bread stuffing	½ cup	20
Breadstick: soft	1 breadstick	15–25
Bun: hamburger or hot dog	1 regular size	15–30
Corn bread	2 cubes	15
Croissant	Medium 2 oz	25
Dinner roll	Small	15
English muffin	1 whole	30
Pancake	6" diameter (avg size)	30
Pita bread	Large 6"–9"	30–45
Tortilla: corn	7"	15
Waffle (frozen type)	1	15

Cereals/Beans/Grains/Pasta	Portion Size	Carbs (g)
Beans: refried	½ cup	18
Oatmeal, cooked	½ cup	10
Cream of Wheat, cooked	½ cup	15
Cornmeal: dry	3 Tbsp	15
Beans/Legumes/Lentils: as prepared	½ cup	15
Flour: dry	3 Tbsp	15
Hummus	½ cup	10–15
Pasta, cooked	1 cup	45
Rice, cooked	1 cup	45

Starchy Vegetables	Portion Size	Carbs (g)
Corn: cooked or canned	½ cup	15
Corn on the cob	6"–9"	30–45
Peas	½ cup	15
Potato: Wendy's	Avg baked (10 oz)	60
Potatoes (hashed, mashed)	½ cup	15
Squash (winter type: acorn, Hubbard, etc)	1 cup	10–30
Sweet Potato/Yams: plain cooked	10 oz baked	60

Milk & Yogurt	Portion Size	Carbs (g)
Cow's milk (fat-free, 1 percent, 2 percent, whole)	1 cup	12
Rice milk: plain	1 cup	20
Soy milk (plain)	1 cup	8
Yogurt (plain)	1 cup	12
Yogurt: Dannon Light & Fit	1 serving (6 oz)	10
Yogurt: Yoplait Light (blue top)	1 serving (6 oz)	19

Fruit	Portion Size	Carbs (g)
Apple	4–8 oz	15–30
Applesauce: unsweetened	½ cup	15
Apricots, dried	7 pieces	15
Banana	6"–9"	30–45
Blackberries, Blueberries	1 cup	20
Fruit Cocktail (canned in its own juice)	½ cup	15
Cantaloupe, Honeydew Melons	1 cup	15
Cherries	12	15
Dates: dried Medjool type	1	15
Grapefruit	½ large	15
Grapes	15 small	15
Kiwi	1 small	15
Orange	1 medium	15
Peaches (canned in their own juice)	½ cup	15
Pear	6 oz	20
Pineapple	1 cup diced	20
Prunes: dried	3	15
Raisins	35 or ⅛ cup (2 Tbsp)	15
Raspberries	1 cup	15
Strawberries: fresh	1 cup halves	12
Watermelon	1 cup diced	12

Fruit/Vegetable Juice	Portion Size	Carbs (g)
Apple juice 100 percent	½ cup	15
Carrot juice	1 cup	12
Cranberry juice cocktail 100 percent	½ cup	12

Cranberry juice cocktail: light	1 cup	10
Grape juice 100 percent	½ cup (4 oz)	15
Orange juice	½ cup	13
Tomato juice/V8	1 cup (8 oz)	10

Baked Goods

Cake, 2 layer, frosted	4″ square	80
Chocolate chip cookie: refrigerator dough	1	15
Danish (large bakery type)	1	45
Donut (Dunkin' Donuts: plain or jelly filled)	1	25–40
Donut (Krispy Kreme)	1	20
Apple crisp	½ cup	70
Fruit pie	⅛ of 9″ pie	50
Muffin (homemade standard size)	1	20–30
Muffins: bakery type	1	60–75

Snack Foods

Dark chocolate	1 oz	15
Dove chocolate	3 pieces	15
French fries: crinkle cut frozen type	10	15
French fries: diner style	Side order	60
French fries: fast food	Small order	30
Graham cracker	3 squares	15
Hershey kisses	5	15
Ice cream: no sugar added	½ cup	12–15
Ice cream: plain vanilla	½ cup	15
Jell-O	½ cup	20

Jell-O: sugar free	½ cup	0
Oyster crackers	½ cup	15
Popcorn	3 cups	15
Potato chips	1 oz (10–15 chips)	15
Pretzels	11 small	15
Pudding: regular	1 snack pack	30
Pudding: sugar free	1 snack pack	15
Saltine crackers	7 squares	15
Sherbet	½ cup	30
Sorbet	½ cup	35–40
Tortilla chips	1 oz (10–15 chips)	20

SUGAR AND DIABETES

Glucose is one of the most important sources of energy for your body. We need sugar to live and function correctly. When we consume sugar and the levels rise in our blood, our body responds by secreting the hormone insulin from our pancreas. Insulin does two important things once it comes in contact with the sugar. Because sugar can't enter most of your cells on its own, insulin attaches to the sugar so that it can be transported into the cells and used as energy. Insulin's next important function is to help the body store excess sugar. If you have more sugar in your body than it needs, insulin will help store the sugar in your liver. This storage form of glucose is called *glycogen*. In between meals or during intense physical activity such as running, when blood sugar levels drop too low and more sugar is needed, the hormone glucagon stimulates your liver to convert the glycogen back to glucose, which then release into your blood to be used as energy.

Type 1 diabetes, the less common form of the two, is caused by the destruction of the cells in the pancreas that make insulin. This form of diabetes typically develops during one's youth but less often can strike during adult years. Those who suffer from type 1 diabetes cannot sufficiently produce enough insulin to handle the rising blood sugar levels after meals. They typically need insulin medications via injections to help control their blood sugar levels.

Type 2 diabetes, the most common form of the two, typically accounts for 90 to 95 percent of all diagnosed cases of diabetes. This type of diabetes typically occurs during adulthood, but with the rising levels of childhood obesity, we are seeing a sharp rise in youth and adolescents developing what was once an adults-only disease. Type 2 diabetes is a matter of the body's cells not responding appropriately to the insulin that the pancreas creates. The body becomes *insulin-resistant*. Unfortunately, as type 2 diabetes gets worse, the pancreas may produce even less insulin. This condition is called *insulin deficiency*. Lifestyle changes such as weight loss, exercise, and proper nutrition, as well as medications that are typically in a pill form (although for severe type 2 diabetics they may require insulin) can help control type 2.

BROWN VERSUS WHITE SUGAR

Brown sugar is simply sugar that contains molasses. It's the molasses that gives it the distinctive brown color and flavor. There are two ways that brown sugar can be made. In the first, the unrefined or partially refined brown sugar still contains some of the original molasses from the cane plant, and it has not all been lost in the refining process. You might find this sugar labeled in several ways: raw, natural, demerara, turbinado, and muscovado. These sugars tend not to be as soft and moist as the refined (processed) brown sugars.

The second way that brown sugar is made is through a process called refinement. Molasses is added back to the refined white sugar. This tends to be the brown sugar you purchase in the store. It's soft and moist, and this is what is commonly referred to as brown sugar. Light brown sugar versus dark brown sugar is simply a matter of molasses content, with the dark brown sugar containing almost double the amount of molasses (6.5 percent vs. 3.5 percent). Despite what many people think, there really isn't any impactful nutritional difference between brown and white sugar, and they tend to be equally sweet.

DANGERS OF TOO MUCH SUGAR

Lots of research has gone into understanding the potential dangers of overconsuming sugar. A plethora of studies strongly suggest that a high intake of added sugar is linked to an increase in body fat, and eventually obesity. Sugar is a form of energy, so when you consume more sugar than your body needs or uses, the extra energy needs to go somewhere—typically that means being converted to triglycerides, a fat that tends to be stored around your waistline, hips, and thighs. Sugary drinks are probably the worst culprits; not only are you consuming excess sugar, but these liquid calories tend not to be satisfying and you are left hungry to consume even more.

Research has also shown that too much sugar can compromise the body's immune system—one of the most important defense mechanisms that the body has to fight infections and other illnesses.

High sugar levels over a prolonged time can actually harm the ever-important pancreas and reduce its ability to make insulin. When sugar levels are too high, the pancreas overcompensates and insulin levels remain too high. Eventually, this leads to the organ being permanently damaged.

Sustained high levels of blood sugar can also cause changes that lead to a hardening of the blood vessels, something called athero-sclerosis. This means that almost any part of the body can be harmed by too much sugar in the bloodstream. Here are just some of the problems that can be caused by damaged blood vessels:

- Strokes
- Heart attacks
- Kidney disease/kidney failure
- Vision loss or blindness
- Erectile dysfunction
- Nerve damage (neuropathy) that causes tingling, pain, or less sensation in your feet, legs, and hands
- Poor circulation to the legs and feet
- Slow wound healing

Reducing sugar in your diet is going to deliver immediate and long-term changes to your health. Living the rest of your life without eating some sugar or carbohydrates is virtually impossible, but being mindful of the sugar content of foods and the dangers of consuming too much sugar can keep you on a path to better weight management and stave off disease.

ARTIFICIAL SWEETENERS AND SUGAR SUBSTITUTES

Walk down any grocery store aisle and you will find products that contain various types of sugar, sugar substitutes, and artificial sweeteners. For most of these products, there is no unanimity in the nutritional and medical community about the safety, effectiveness, and overall general use guidelines for these products. Here is a list of some common sugar substitutes and artificial sweeteners.

Agave Nectar

This natural sweetener derives from the agave cactus and has a taste and texture quite similar to honey. It contains about 20 calories per teaspoon—almost as much as honey—but doesn't contain the same amount of beneficial antioxidants and other phytonutrients. Agave is sweeter tasting than sugar, so it requires less to get the same sweetness. Agave contains more fructose than table sugar, which means it's less likely to cause a blood sugar spike—something we are trying to avoid. This benefit, unfortunately, could be offset by the possibility that it's more likely to reduce your sensitivity to insulin and lower your metabolism.

Aspartame

This is one of the world's most studied artificial sweeteners and can commonly be found in the popular brands such as Equal and Nutra Sweet. Approved by the U.S. Food and Drug Administration (FDA) in 1981, aspartame contains no calories, which has made it a darling of the diet industry. There have been many charges levied against this sweetener, from weight gain to immune system dysfunction to cancer. Several large organizations such as the FDA, American Dietetic Association, and World Health Organization find that it poses no threat in moderation. However, the Center for Science in the Public Interest gave it their lowest ranking when reviewing food additives. One thing that almost everyone agrees on is that people with phenylketonuria—a rare inherited genetic disorder that causes the amino acid phenylalanine to build up in your body—should avoid it.

High-Fructose Corn Syrup

One of the most controversial sweeteners on the market, high-fructose corn syrup is typically found in sodas, sauces, cereals, and desserts. It contains fructose and glucose and is derived from processed corn syrup. It weighs in at 17 calories per teaspoon, and manufacturers like to use it in their products because it's cheaper than table sugar and gives products a longer shelf life. The jury is out about whether it's as contributory to obesity as many believe, but most nutritionists and health advocates recommend eliminating it from your diet altogether or severely restricting the amount that you consume.

Honey

This natural sweetener contains trace amounts of vitamins and minerals and contains approximately 21 calories per teaspoon compared to the 16 calories found in table sugar. Studies suggest, however, that it may not raise blood sugar as fast as other sweeteners, which is important because it's better for the body to have a slow, steady rise in blood sugar after eating rather than a dramatic spike.

Stevia Leaf Extract

Stevia is considered an alternative to artificial sweeteners. It is a product derived naturally from the stevia plant and is also called *rebiana*. Stevia doesn't contain any calories. Refined stevia products gained a "generally recommended as safe" approval from the FDA in

2008. In 2013, the Center for Science in the Public Interest deemed it to be safe, although deserving of better testing. All stevia is not created equally, so you should be aware of whether the product is highly processed. The more the stevia is processed, the less of a true product it is, so be cautious when choosing these products.

Sucralose

This is an artificial sweetener commonly found under the brand name Splenda. Approved in 1998 by the FDA, Splenda has remained controversial. It is not heat sensitive, so it can be used in baking. Many diabetics and those looking to keep their blood sugar in control use it because it contains no calories or carbs. Most credible studies find it to be safe and not cancer causing, although one study showed that it might have a negative impact on the immune system.

Sucrose

This is what we consider to be table sugar. With 16 calories per teaspoon, sucrose is naturally found in fruit and typically added to baked goods, salad dressings, jelly, and other products. There are no nutritional benefits offered by sucrose, although anyone who has been around a child who has consumed a large amount of sugar can attest that it does temporarily increase energy levels. It causes a sharp rise of blood sugar, which is something that we should try to avoid.

3 WEEK 1: CALIBRATION

This is the beginning of the new you. This week is the first week of your new life. Embrace the changes and know that they are going to improve the quality and length of your life. You will never eat or exercise perfectly, but you can find a rhythm that answers the need to make improvements and at the same time bring you pleasure and a sense of normalcy. The first step in forming the new you is calibrating—planning and preparing the way you eat and move so that it's critical to your success. Take a few minutes and look through what the week has in store for you, then make sure your meals are planned at least three days in advance so that you have the foods and snacks available to you when needed or that you know where and when you can get them. Try to choose a variety of foods and not always have the same meal for breakfast or lunch. If you need to swap days because you have better access to foods on one day than you do another, feel free to do so. Otherwise, try your best to stick to the plan and deviate only if you have an allergy, a severe dislike of an item, or the food is a known trigger that you should avoid.

Note: When the meal plan calls for maple syrup, please note that people metabolize sugar differently, so instead of the 100 percent maple syrup you might try sugar-free syrup. This is a determination that you need to make. There are a lot of carbs in maple syrup, so you need to be very mindful of not consuming too much, especially if your blood sugars are sensitive. Also, when bread is allowed, you can substitute sprouted bread for the suggested 100% whole-wheat or 100% whole-grain bread.

BAD HABIT _____

CHANGE _____

GOOD HABIT _____

IMPROVABLE HABIT _____

CHANGE _____

WEEK 1, DAY 1

BREAKFAST

Choose one main dish:

- 1 or 2 scrambled eggs cooked in olive oil or cooking spray, salt and pepper to taste
- 1 cup of cold cereal, not sugar-coated, with ½ cup of skim, or reduced-fat milk

Power Ups:

- 2 slices of 100% whole-grain or 100% whole-wheat toast
- ½ cup of fresh strawberries, sliced

SNACK

- 10–20 grams of carbohydrates (e.g., ¼ cup of dried fruit and nut mix or 1 cup of chicken noodle soup, tomato soup—made with water—or vegetable soup). For a list of snack options, see chapter 8.

LUNCH

Choose one main dish:

- ½ cup tuna salad in a 100% whole-grain or 100% whole-wheat pita
- 1 cup of lentil soup, bean soup, or vegetable soup and 1 small salad with 2 tablespoons of fat-free, light salad dressing

> **— NUTRI NUGGET —**
> Fiber can help prevent blood sugar spikes. Research has shown that a diet that contains a healthy amount of fiber can lower your risk of diabetes and heart disease by as much as 20–30 percent.
> *Source: American Diabetes Assoc.*

SNACK

- 10–20 grams of carbohydrates

DINNER

Choose one main dish:

- 6 ounces of fish (salmon, halibut, tuna, trout), grilled/baked (NOT fried)
- 1 beef burrito (if frozen choose low sodium and carbohydrate count less than 35) with beans and 1 tablespoon of cheese
- Spinach Fusilli with Roasted Mushrooms (recipe page 185)

Power Ups:

- 2 servings of vegetables

SNACK

- Fewer than 10 grams of carbohydrates

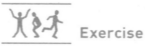 Exercise

Below and on subsequent days, you will find a suggested time and type of exercise. For a more detailed description of these exercises, go to pages 209–212 and read about the best way to perform them.

- 20 minutes: Cardiovascular/aerobic activity in the morning
- 15 minutes: Cardiovascular/aerobic activity in the late afternoon/evening

WEEK 1, DAY 2

BREAKFAST

Choose one main dish:

- 86-ounce fruit smoothie with no sugar or other sweeteners added
- 1 slice of french toast with 1 teaspoon of 100% maple syrup
- Egg and Veggie Breakfast Sandwich (recipe page 123)

Power Ups:

- If you choose the smoothie, you can also have 2 slices of 100% whole-grain or 100% whole-wheat toast with a small amount of butter or sugar-free jelly spread
- If you choose the french toast, you can also have ½ cup of berries

SNACK

- 10–20 grams of carbohydrates

LUNCH

Choose one main dish:

- Chicken sandwich on 2 slices of 100% whole-grain or 100% whole-wheat toast with lettuce, tomato, and 1 teaspoon of mayonnaise or mustard
- Turkey sandwich on 2 slices of 100% whole-grain or 100% whole-wheat toast with lettuce, tomato, and 1 teaspoon of mayonnaise or mustard
- Curry Chicken Skewers (recipe page 133)

Power Ups:

- ½ cup of raw vegetables (e.g., carrots, cucumbers, celery)

SNACK
- 10–20 grams of carbohydrates

DINNER

Choose one main dish:
- 5 ounces of herb-roasted turkey
- 4 ounces of boneless pork chops, grilled/baked, trimmed of fat

Power Ups:
- ½ cup of steamed or grilled cauliflower or other vegetable
- ½ cup of cooked brown rice

SNACK
- Fewer than 10 grams of carbohydrates

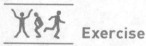 **Exercise**

- 30 minutes: Cardiovascular/aerobic activity
- 15 minutes: Resistance training

WEEK 1, DAY 3

BREAKFAST

Choose one main dish:

- Omelet with diced vegetables
- ½ of a two-inch bran muffin with ¼ cup of sliced fresh berries and 2 tablespoons of low-fat or nonfat yogurt

Power Ups:

- 1 medium apple
- 1 slice of 100% whole-grain or 100% whole-wheat toast with 1 teaspoon of butter or sugar-free jelly spread

SNACK

- 10–20 grams of carbohydrates

LUNCH

Choose one main dish:

- 1 cup tomato soup or black bean soup (without cream)
- Medium green garden salad (2 cups of greens with tomatoes, olives, shaved carrots, cucumbers) with 2 tablespoons of fat-free, light salad dressing

Power Ups:

- 1 piece of medium-sized fruit or ½ cup of berries

SNACK

- 10–20 grams of carbohydrates

NUTRI NUGGET

A typical 20 oz soda contains 15–18 teaspoons of sugar and upwards of 240 calories.
Source: Harvard School of Public Health

DINNER

Choose one main dish:

- 6 ounces of grilled/baked chicken breast with roasted lemon
- Chicken stir-fry (use 6 ounces of chicken, low-sodium soy sauce, and 1 cup of veggies)

Power Ups:

- 1 cup of vegetables
- ½ cup of cooked brown rice

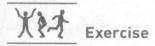 **Exercise**

REST DAY!

WEEK 1, DAY 4

BREAKFAST

Choose one main dish:

- 1 cup of oatmeal or Cream of Wheat with ½ cup of skim or reduced-fat milk
- 1 breakfast burrito (scrambled egg, bell pepper, and onion in a warm 100% whole-wheat or 100% whole-grain tortilla, sprinkled with 1 tablespoon of salsa and 1 tablespoon of shredded nonfat cheese)

Power Ups:

- 1 piece of medium-sized fruit

SNACK

- 10–20 grams of carbohydrates

LUNCH

Choose one main dish:

- ¼ pound hamburger with optional ketchup and mustard and 1 small portion of french fries with ketchup (1 teaspoon), along with 1 small green garden salad with 1 tablespoon of fat-free, light salad dressing
- Caesar salad with grilled chicken (total weight 12 ounces) with 2 tablespoons of fat-free, light salad dressing
- Barley with Grapefruit, Spinach, and Almonds (recipe page 180)

Power Ups:

- 1 piece of medium-sized fruit

SNACK

- 10–20 grams of carbohydrates

DINNER

Choose one main dish:

- 5 ounces of fish, grilled
- 5 ounces of shrimp, grilled/baked

Power Ups:

- 1 cup of vegetables (you can have ½ cup of one vegetable and ½ cup of another)
- 1 cup of cooked brown rice

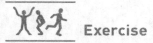 **Exercise**

- 35 minutes: Cardiovascular/aerobic activity

WEEK 1, DAY 5

BREAKFAST

Choose one main dish:

- 1 cup of whole-grain, high-fiber cereal with ½ cup skim or reduced-fat milk
- ½ whole-grain bagel spread with 1 tablespoon of light cream cheese and 1 teaspoon of a low-sugar fruit spread
- The Honey Buzz smoothie (recipe page 199)

Power Ups:

- If you choose the smoothie, no Power Ups. For other main dishes, choose all or none below.
- 1 cup of berries
- 1 slice of 100% whole-grain or 100% whole-wheat toast with 1 teaspoon of butter or sugar-free jelly spread (only if you choose the cereal option)

SNACK

- 10–20 grams of carbohydrates

LUNCH

Choose one main dish:

- Tuna sandwich (2 slices of 100% whole-grain or 100% whole-wheat bread, ½ cup of tuna, water-packed, 1 tablespoon of mayonnaise, 1 teaspoon of diced onion, 1 tablespoon of diced celery, 1 teaspoon of relish)

> **— NUTRI NUGGET —**
>
> People who consume sugary drinks regularly—1 to 2 cans a day or more—have a 26 percent greater risk of developing type 2 diabetes than people who rarely have such drinks.
> *Source: Diabetes Care. 2010;33:2477–83*

- Steak sandwich with 5 ounces of lean steak on whole-wheat roll with ½ slice of melted nonfat cheese, and ¼ cup of peppers and ¼ cup of diced onion (optional)

Power Ups:
- 1 small piece of fruit
- 1 cup of vegetables, raw or cooked

SNACK
- 10–20 grams of carbohydrates

DINNER
Choose one main dish:
- Large green garden salad with diced chicken and 2 tablespoons of fat-free, light salad dressing

Power Ups:
- 1 medium baked sweet potato
- 1 ounce of grated reduced- or low-fat cheese

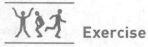 **Exercise**

- 30 minutes: Cardiovascular/aerobic activity
- 25 minutes: Resistance training

WEEK 1, DAY 6

BREAKFAST

Choose one main dish:

- 2 scrambled eggs with 1 tablespoon of melted nonfat or reduced-fat cheddar cheese, cooked in oil or cooking spray
- 6 ounces of fat-free, light plain yogurt with ¼ cup of granola, ¼ cup of blueberries, and 1 tablespoon of chopped nuts, if desired

Power Ups:

- 1 slice of 100% whole-grain or 100% whole-wheat toast
- 1 cup of berries

SNACK

- 10–20 grams of carbohydrates

LUNCH

Choose one main dish:

- 1 cup of pasta and bean soup
- 1 all-beef hot dog (6 inches), with 1 teaspoon of mustard, 1 teaspoon of ketchup, and ½ teaspoon of relish, if desired, on whole-wheat bun

Power Ups:

- ½ cup of raw vegetables
- 1 slice of 100% whole-grain or 100% whole-wheat bread (only if you choose the soup option)
- 4 onion rings, no bigger than 3 inches across

SNACK

- 10–20 grams of carbohydrates

DINNER

Choose one main dish:

- Grilled or steamed shrimp (6–8 pieces) with a tablespoon of butter or other sauce
- 5-ounce slice of meat loaf made from lean beef with tomato sauce

Power Ups:

- ½ cup of cooked brown rice
- ½ cup of green beans

SNACK

- Fewer than 10 grams of carbohydrates

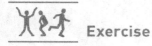 Exercise

REST DAY!

WEEK 1, DAY 7

BREAKFAST

Choose one main dish:

- 12-ounce fruit smoothie (25 grams of carbs or fewer), such as Antioxidant Supreme (recipe page 201)
- 2 whole-wheat pancakes, measuring 5 inches across, with 1 teaspoon of butter and 1 teaspoon of 100 percent maple syrup

Power Ups:

- If you choose the smoothie, no Power Ups.
- If you choose the pancakes: 100% whole-grain or 100% whole-wheat English muffin with 1 teaspoon low-sugar jelly spread

SNACK

- 10–20 grams of carbohydrates

LUNCH

Choose one main dish:

- 1 slice of cheese pizza with medium-sized green garden salad with 2 tablespoons of fat-free, light salad dressing
- 1 turkey burger with 1 slice of fat-free cheese, lettuce, tomato, and 1 teaspoon of mayonnaise and 1 teaspoon of ketchup

---

NUTRI NUGGET

Type 2 diabetes is largely preventable. About 9 cases in 10 could be avoided by taking several simple steps: keeping weight under control, exercising more, eating a healthy diet, and not smoking.

Source: Harvard School of Public Health

Power Ups:
- 1 cup of sliced carrot sticks and 2 tablespoons of hummus
- 1 cup of plain air-popped popcorn

SNACK
- 10–20 grams of carbohydrates

DINNER
Choose one main dish:
- Grilled/baked chicken or grilled/baked pork chop
- 5 ounces of fish, grilled/baked

Power Ups:
- ½ cup of steamed broccoli
- ½ cup of mashed sweet potatoes (use fat-free buttermilk instead of cream, and unsalted butter)

SNACK
- Fewer than 10 grams of carbohydrates

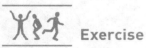 Exercise

- 20 minutes: Cardiovascular/aerobic activity
- 15 minutes: Resistance training

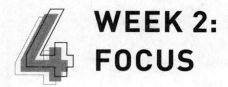

WEEK 2: FOCUS

Your first week is in the rearview mirror and now you are on to week 2. This is a week all about focus and commitment. Many people can get through the first week of many programs, but it's during week 2 that many start to stumble. Doubts start to seep in. Temptation to stray away from the program increases. Second-guessing starts to overcome your initial excitement and confidence. This is why week 2 is your week of *focus*.

This week will include more tasty food options and will continue to reduce the amount of unhealthy sugars that you consume and increase the amount of good carbohydrates. You might experience some sugar cravings if you were consuming high levels of sugar before starting the program. This is normal and you should not be alarmed. Focus yourself this week on your transformation and on your new, healthier way of eating and moving and you will enjoy the journey.

BAD HABIT _____

CHANGE _____

GOOD HABIT _____

IMPROVABLE HABIT _____

CHANGE _____

WEEK 2, DAY 1

BREAKFAST

Choose one main dish:
- 1 egg, scrambled
- 1 cup of whole-grain breakfast cereal, hot or cold with skim or reduced-fat milk

Power Ups:
- 1 cup skim or reduced-fat milk
- 1 piece of medium-sized fruit
- Water (unlimited), 1 cup of tea or 1 cup of black coffee with 1 tablespoon of low-calorie cream, or ½ cup of fresh juice

SNACK
- 10–20 grams of carbohydrates

LUNCH

Choose one main dish:
- Grilled chicken with lettuce and tomato on 100% whole-grain or 100% whole-wheat toast with 1 teaspoon of mayonnaise or mustard
- Roast beef sandwich on 100% whole-grain or 100% whole-wheat bread, with 1 teaspoon of mayonnaise or mustard and 1 slice of fat-free or reduced-fat cheese
- Turkey-Quinoa Burgers (recipe page 145)

> **NUTRI NUGGET**
>
> Fiber is a type of carbohydrate, but unlike other carbs, the body can't digest it. Though most carbohydrates are broken down into sugar molecules, fiber cannot be broken down, so instead it passes through the body undigested. Fiber is important in the body's sugar regulation by helping to keep hunger and blood sugar in check.

Power Ups:
- ½ cup of raw vegetables

SNACK
- 10–20 grams of carbohydrates

DINNER
Choose one main dish:
- 5 ounces of fish, grilled/baked
- 2½ × 4-inch slice of meat lasagna

Power Ups:
- ½ cup of cooked brown rice
- ½ cup of broccoli

SNACK
- Fewer than 10 grams of carbohydrates

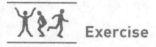 Exercise

- 35 minutes: Cardiovascular/aerobic activity

WEEK 2, DAY 2

BREAKFAST
Choose one main dish:
- 2 pancakes (4½ inches across) with 1 tablespoon of 100 percent maple syrup
- 1 croissant with 1 egg, 1 slice of reduced-fat cheese, and 1 slice bacon
- Breakfast Grits with Oranges and Pecans (recipe page 120)

Power Ups:
- ½ large grapefruit or 8 melon balls or a quarter slice of a small melon

SNACK
- 10–20 grams of carbohydrates

LUNCH
Choose one main dish:
- Turkey wrap in a whole-wheat pita with 4 ounces of turkey and lettuce, tomato, and fat-free, light salad dressing
- 1 cup of chicken noodle soup

Power Ups:
- ½ cup of vegetables
- 8 small whole-wheat crackers

SNACK
- 10–20 grams of carbohydrates

DINNER
Choose one main dish:
- 1 cup of whole-wheat spaghetti with four small 1-inch meatballs in marinara sauce
- 5 ounces of skinless, boneless chicken, grilled/baked

Power Ups:
- 1 cup of vegetables divided into 2 types (e.g., ½ cup squash and ½ cup carrots)

SNACK
- Fewer than 10 grams of carbohydrates

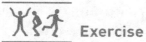 **Exercise**

- 35 minutes: Cardiovascular/aerobic activity
- 20 minutes: Resistance exercises

WEEK 2, DAY 3

BREAKFAST

Choose one main dish:

- 1 yogurt parfait (1 cup of fat-free, low-calorie plain yogurt with ½ cup fresh fruit)
- 1 cup of oatmeal with ½ cup skim or reduced-fat milk, ½ teaspoon of honey, and 1 teaspoon of butter, if desired

Power Ups:

- 1 slice of whole-grain toast with ½ teaspoon of sugar-free jelly spread

SNACK

- 10–20 grams of carbohydrates

LUNCH

Choose one main dish:

- Grilled chicken salad (2 cups mixed greens mixed with 3 ounces of skinless diced chicken, ⅓ cup of chopped bell pepper, ⅓ cup of chopped onion, 5 cherry tomatoes, ⅓ cup of shredded carrot, and 2 tablespoons of fat-free, light salad dressing)

NUTRI NUGGET

Added sugars are sugars and syrups that are added to foods or beverages during processing or preparation. They do not include naturally occurring sugars such as those found in milk (lactose) and fruits (fructose). Added sugars (or added sweeteners) include natural sugars (such as white sugar, brown sugar, and honey) as well as other caloric sweeteners that are chemically manufactured (such as high-fructose corn syrup). Some names for added sugars include agave syrup, brown sugar, corn sweetener, corn syrup, sugar molecules ending in "ose" (dextrose, fructose, glucose, lactose, maltose, sucrose), high-fructose corn syrup, fruit juice concentrate, honey, invert sugar, malt sugar, molasses, raw sugar, sugar, syrup.

Source: American Heart Association

- Ham and cheese sandwich (4 ounces ham on 2 slices of 100% whole-wheat or 100% whole-grain bread with 1 slice of low-fat or reduced-fat cheese, 1 teaspoon of mayonnaise or mustard)

Power Ups:
- Herb-Crusted Beefsteak Tomatoes (recipe page 179)
- 1 small apple
- Six ¼-inch-thick cucumber slices with 1 teaspoon of fat-free, light salad dressing for dipping

SNACK
- 10–20 grams of carbohydrates

DINNER
Choose one main dish:
- 5 ounces of fish, grilled/baked
- 1 cup of beef stew

Power Ups:
- 1 whole-grain roll (2×2 inches)
- ½ cup of cooked brown rice

SNACK
- Fewer than 10 grams of carbohydrates

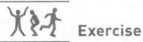 **Exercise**

REST DAY!

WEEK 2, DAY 4

BREAKFAST

Choose one main dish:

- 1 fresh peach sliced with ½ cup of low-fat, low-sodium cottage cheese
- 1 cup of hot cooked cereal with ½ cup of skim or reduced-fat milk

Power Ups:

- ¾ cup fresh blueberries or sliced strawberries

SNACK

- 10–20 grams of carbohydrates

LUNCH

Choose one main dish:

- Tuna melt (1 toasted whole-grain English muffin topped with ⅓ cup of tuna mixed with 1 tablespoon of light mayonnaise, 1 teaspoon of relish, and 1 ounce of fat-free or reduced-fat cheese)
- Chicken salad (2 cups of mixed greens, ¼ cup of sliced red grapes, 3 ounces of cooked chicken breast, 6 slices of cucumbers, 1 stalk of chopped celery, optional, and drizzled with 2 tablespoons of fat-free, light salad dressing)

Power Ups:

- 1 small piece of fruit

SNACK

- 10–20 grams of carbohydrates

DINNER

Choose one main dish:

- Egg and Spinach Frittata
- 1 cup of whole-wheat spaghetti with meat sauce

Power Ups:

- 1 cup of steamed or grilled vegetables
- 1 small 100% whole-grain or whole-wheat roll

SNACK

- Fewer than 10 grams of carbohydrates

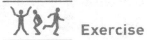 Exercise

- 35 minutes: Cardiovascular/aerobic activity

WEEK 2, DAY 5

BREAKFAST

Choose one main dish:
- 1 egg, scrambled with 1 ounce of fat-free or reduced-fat cheese, cooked in oil or cooking spray
- 1 cup of cold cereal, no sugar added, with ½ cup of low-fat, fat-free, or reduced-fat milk

Power Ups:
- 1 small orange or banana
- 2 slices of 100% whole-grain or whole-wheat bread or one 100% whole-grain or whole-wheat English muffin

SNACK
- 10–20 grams of carbohydrates

LUNCH

Choose one main dish:
- Roast beef sandwich (3 ounces of lean roast beef, lettuce, and slice of tomato on 2 slices of 100% whole-grain or 100% whole-wheat bread, with 1 teaspoon of mayonnaise or mustard)
- 1 cup vegetable soup topped with 1 teaspoon of nonfat plain yogurt and 5 halved cherry tomatoes
- Classic Cucumber Gazpacho (recipe page 146)

Power Ups:
- 1 small green garden salad with 1 tablespoon of fat-free, light salad dressing

SNACK

- 10–20 grams of carbohydrates

DINNER

Choose one main dish:

- Barbecue chicken (4 ounces of chicken tender strips or 2 drumsticks with 2 tablespoons of barbecue sauce)
- Tofu stir-fry (4 ounces of tofu, with 2 cups of mixed veggies cooked in 2 tablespoons of low-sodium stir-fry sauce and 1 tablespoon of olive oil; served over 1 cup of cooked brown rice)

Power Ups:

- ½ cup of cooked cabbage
- ½ cup of mashed sweet potatoes (use fat-free buttermilk instead of cream, and unsalted butter)

SNACK

- Fewer than 10 grams of carbohydrates

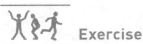 **Exercise**

- 30 minutes: Cardiovascular/aerobic activity
- 25 minutes: Resistance exercises

NUTRI NUGGET

According to new USDA guidelines, sugar should be limited to 10 percent or less of a person's daily calories. For example, if you consume 2000 calories in a day, you should not consume more than 200 calories in the form of sugar.

Source: USDA

WEEK 2, DAY 6

BREAKFAST
Choose one main dish:
- 12-ounce fruit smoothie (250 calories or less and 30 grams of carbs or fewer)
- 1 whole-grain or whole-wheat waffle (5 inches in diameter) with 1 teaspoon 100 percent maple syrup

Power Ups:
- 2 strips of pork or turkey bacon

SNACK
- 10–20 grams of carbohydrates

LUNCH
Choose one main dish:
- 1 whole-wheat tortilla chicken wrap (4 ounces of chicken, 1 teaspoon of hummus, ½ cup of mixed greens, 1 teaspoon of fat-free or reduced-fat cheese, and ¼ cup of sun-dried tomatoes, optional)
- 1 cup of vegetable chili

Power Ups:
- 1 cup of cooked brown rice

SNACK
- 10–20 grams of carbohydrates

DINNER
Choose one main dish:
- 5 ounces of salmon or other fish, grilled/baked

- 1 Caesar salad with chicken
- Golden Carrot Soup (recipe page 175)

Power Ups:
- 1 cup of cooked brown or wild rice
- 1 cup of steamed summer squash

SNACK
- Fewer than 10 grams of carbohydrates

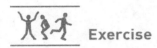 Exercise

REST DAY!

WEEK 2, DAY 7

BREAKFAST

Choose one main dish:
- Grilled cheese sandwich on 2 slices of 100% whole-grain or whole-wheat bread
- 8-ounce yogurt parfait with granola and fruit

Power Ups:
- 1 small piece of fruit

SNACK
- 10–20 grams of carbohydrates

LUNCH

Choose one main dish:
- Veggie cheeseburger on 100% whole-grain or 100% whole-wheat bun
- Tuna salad sandwich on 100% whole-grain or 100% whole-wheat bread

Power Ups:
- 1 cup of berries or 1 small piece of fruit

SNACK
- 10–20 grams of carbohydrates

DINNER

Choose one main dish:
- 5 ounces of pan-seared steak

NUTRI NUGGET

Drinking one can of soda per day can increase your risk of dying from heart disease by almost 33 percent.
Source: Journal of the American Medical Association Intern Med. 2014;174(4):516–524.

- 1½ cups of chicken stir-fry
- Hearty Vegetable Stew (recipe page 176)

Power Ups:
- 1 cup of vegetable medley (only if you selected the steak or chicken stir-fry)
- ½ cup of cauliflower, raw, cooked, or steamed

SNACK
- Fewer than 10 grams of carbohydrates

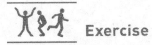 Exercise

- 35 minutes: Cardiovascular/aerobic activity

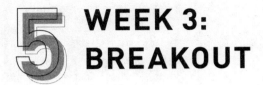

WEEK 3: BREAKOUT

Welcome to week 3! You will continue to eat flavor-ful, satisfying food but not be controlled by the erratic undulations of sugar spikes and troughs. This is your breakout week: You now have two weeks under your belt, and this new way of eating and moving is starting to gel into a lifestyle that you can enjoy and maintain without stress and the feeling of being overly restricted.

It's important to continue to consider habits—both good and bad—that can be changed, enhanced, or stopped. We're always a work in progress, and taking this mental approach allows you to try new things yet not be too disappointed if you fail. Take a little time to think about what your day's activity and meal schedule are going to be. Just five minutes of mental preparation can prevent you from making poor decisions that can throw you off plan. Not only should you be feeling and looking better, but your confidence should be noticeably on the rise!

BAD HABIT _____

CHANGE _____

GOOD HABIT _____

IMPROVABLE HABIT _____

CHANGE _____

WEEK 3, DAY 1

BREAKFAST

Choose one main dish:

- 2 scrambled eggs with diced veggies
- 1 cup of oatmeal with ½ cup skim or reduced-fat milk, ½ teaspoon of honey, and ½ teaspoon of butter, if desired

NUTRI NUGGET

Soda and sports drinks are the largest food group sources of added sugars (34.4 percent), followed by grain desserts (12.7 percent), fruit drinks (8 percent), candy (6.7 percent), and dairy desserts (5.6 percent).
Source: National and Nutrition Examination Survey (NHANES) spanning period 2003–2010.

Power Ups:

- 1 piece of medium-sized fruit
- Water (unlimited), 1 cup of tea or 1 cup of black coffee with 1 tablespoon of low-calorie cream, or ½ cup of fresh juice

SNACK

- 10–20 grams of carbohydrates

LUNCH

Choose one main dish:

- Grilled chicken salad (2 cups mixed greens mixed with 3 ounces of skinless diced chicken, ⅓ cup of chopped bell pepper, ⅓ cup of chopped onion, 5 cherry tomatoes, ⅓ cup of shredded carrot, and 2 tablespoons of fat-free, light salad dressing)
- Turkey burger on 100% whole-grain or 100% whole-wheat bun

Power Ups:

- 1 serving of vegetables, if you choose the turkey burger

SNACK

- 10–20 grams of carbohydrates

DINNER

Choose one main dish:

- 5 ounces of grilled/baked chicken, or grilled/baked pork chop
- 5 ounces of fish, grilled/baked
- Garlic-Herb Marinated London Broil (recipe page 159)

Power Ups:

- 2 servings of vegetables
- 1 whole-wheat roll
- ½ cup of cooked brown rice or whole-wheat couscous

SNACK

- 10–20 grams of carbohydrates

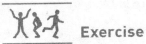 Exercise

- 20 minutes: Cardiovascular/aerobic activity
- 20 minutes: Resistance exercises

WEEK 3, DAY 2

BREAKFAST

Choose one main dish:

- 1 cup of cold cereal, not sugar-coated, with ½ cup of skim or reduced-fat milk
- 1 breakfast burrito (scrambled egg, bell pepper, and onion in a warm, 100% whole-grain or 100% whole-wheat tortilla, sprinkled with 1 tablespoon of salsa and 1 tablespoon of shredded nonfat cheese)
- 6 ounces of fat-free, nonfat plain yogurt with ¼ cup granola, ¼ cup of blueberries, and 1 tablespoon of chopped nuts, if desired

Power Ups:

- 1 piece of medium-sized fruit
- Water (unlimited), 1 cup of tea or 1 cup of black coffee with 1 tablespoon of low-calorie cream, or ½ cup of fresh juice

SNACK

- 10–20 grams of carbohydrates

LUNCH

Choose one main dish:

- 1 slice of cheese pizza and a medium-sized green garden salad with 2 tablespoons of fat-free, light salad dressing
- 1 all-beef hot dog (6 inches) with 1 teaspoon of mustard, 1 teaspoon of ketchup, and ½ teaspoon of relish, if desired, on whole-wheat bun

Power Ups:
- ½ cup of berries or 1 piece of medium-sized fruit
- ½ cup of cooked brown rice

SNACK
- 10–20 grams of carbohydrates

DINNER
Choose one main dish:
- 2 small baked pork chops
- 5 ounces of chicken, grilled/baked with herbs
- 1 cup of whole-wheat pasta with marinara sauce

Power Ups:
- 2 servings of vegetables
- 1 whole-wheat dinner roll

SNACK
- 10–20 grams of carbohydrates

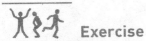 Exercise

REST DAY!

WEEK 3, DAY 3

BREAKFAST
Choose one main dish:
- ¾ cup oatmeal or Cream of Wheat, add ¼ cup of nuts and ground cinnamon for taste, optional
- 12-ounce fruit smoothie (300 calories or less, no sugar or other sweeteners added)

Power Ups:
- 1 piece of medium-sized fruit if you choose the oatmeal, or slice the fruit on top of your cereal
- Water (unlimited), 1 cup of tea or 1 cup of black coffee with 1 tablespoon of low-calorie cream, 1 cup of skim or reduced-fat milk, or ½ cup of fresh juice

SNACK
- 10–20 grams of carbohydrates

LUNCH
Choose one main dish:
- 1 cup of bean soup (kidney, cannellini, or black)
- 5-ounce slice of meat loaf made from lean beef and tomato sauce
- Turkey burger with 1 slice of fat-free cheese, lettuce, tomato, and 1 teaspoon of mayonnaise and 1 teaspoon of ketchup

Power Ups:
- 2 servings of vegetables

SNACK
- 10–20 grams of carbohydrates

DINNER

Choose one main dish:

- 1½ cups of reduced-sodium (less than 480 mg/serving) soup
- 5 ounces of shrimp, grilled/baked
- Grilled Beef Eye Round Steaks with Red Pepper Relish (recipe page 160)

Power Ups:

- 2 servings of vegetables

SNACK

- 10–20 grams of carbohydrates

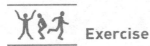 Exercise

- 35 minutes: Cardiovascular/aerobic activity

NUTRI NUGGET

The American Heart Association (AHA) recommends no more than 6 teaspoons (24 grams) of added sugar per day for women and 9 teaspoons (36 grams) for men. The limits for children vary depending on their age and caloric needs, but range between 3–6 teaspoons (12–25 grams) per day.
Source: American Heart Association

WEEK 3, DAY 4

BREAKFAST

Choose one main dish:

- 1 scrambled egg with diced onion, bell pepper, and tomato
- 1 cup of cold cereal, not sugar-coated, with ½ cup of skim or reduced-fat milk
- Tomato-Asparagus Breakfast Casserole (recipe page 116)

Power Ups:

- 100% whole-grain English muffin spread with 2 tablespoons of cottage cheese or 1 teaspoon of butter
- Water (unlimited), 1 cup of tea or 1 cup of black coffee with 1 tablespoon of low-calorie cream, or ½ cup of fresh juice

SNACK

- 10–20 grams of carbohydrates

LUNCH

Choose one main dish:

- Grilled chicken sandwich with lettuce and tomato on 100% whole-grain or 100% whole-wheat toast with 1 teaspoon of light mayonnaise and mustard
- 1 cup of chicken noodle soup
- Roast beef sandwich on 100% whole-grain or whole-wheat bread, with 1 teaspoon of mayonnaise or mustard and 1 slice of fat-free or reduced-fat cheese

Power Ups:

- 1 piece of medium-sized fruit

SNACK

- 10–20 grams of carbohydrates

DINNER

Choose one main dish:

- Vegetarian plate of 3 servings of vegetables
- 1½ cups chicken stir-fry (use 5 ounces of chicken and 1 cup of vegetables)
- 2½ × 4-inch slice meat lasagna

Power Ups:

- 1 serving of vegetables, if you choose the meat to meat lasagna
- ½ cup of cooked brown or dirty rice
- 1 slice of 100% whole-grain bread

SNACK

- 10–20 grams of carbohydrates

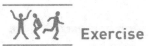 Exercise

- 20 minutes: Cardiovascular/aerobic activity
- 15 minutes: Resistance exercises

NUTRI NUGGET

While diet soda has no calories, it has lots of artificial sweeteners that have been controversial at best. A nine-year study found that older adults who drank diet soda continued to increase their amount of belly fat. Other studies have found that each daily diet soda increases your chance of becoming obese in the next decade by 65 percent. *Diabetes Care* published a study that found drinking diet soft drinks was associated with an increased risk of developing the metabolic syndrome—obesity, high blood pressure, high triglycerides—which lead to diabetes and heart disease.

Source: Sharon P.G. Fowler, Ken Williams, and Helen P. Hazuda. "Diet Soda Intake Is Associated with Long-Term Increases in Waist Circumference in a Biethnic Cohort of Older Adults: The San Antonio Longitudinal Study of Aging." Journal of the American Geriatrics Society, March 17, 2015 DOI: 10.1111/jgs.13376

WEEK 3, DAY 5

BREAKFAST

Choose one main dish:

- Omelet with diced vegetables
- 1 cup of oatmeal or Cream of Wheat with ½ cup of skim or reduced-fat milk

Power Ups:

- 1 slice of 100% whole-wheat or whole-grain toast
- ½ cup of fresh berries
- Water (unlimited), 1 cup of tea or 1 cup of black coffee with 1 tablespoon of low-calorie cream, or ½ cup of fresh juice

SNACK

- 10–20 grams of carbohydrates

LUNCH

Choose one main dish:

- Tuna salad sandwich on 100% whole-grain bread (3–4 ounces of water-packed tuna with celery and 1 tablespoon of mayonnaise)
- 1 all-beef hot dog (6 inches) with 1 teaspoon of mustard, 1 teaspoon of ketchup, and ½ teaspoon of relish, if desired, on whole-wheat bun
- 1 cup of lentil soup or bean soup with 1 small salad with 2 tablespoons of fat-free, light salad dressing
- Turkey Waldorf Salad (recipe page 140)

Power Ups:
- 10 baby carrots with hummus or 1 serving of vegetables

SNACK
- 10–20 grams of carbohydrates

DINNER
Choose one main dish:
- Large tossed salad with greens, tomatoes, shaved carrots, cucumbers, and olives, with 2 tablespoons of fat-free, light salad dressing (3 ounces diced chicken, optional)
- 5 ounces of fish, grilled/baked
- 5 ounces of steak, grilled

Power Ups:
- 2 servings of vegetables, if you choose the fish or steak
- 1 whole-wheat roll for all entrée choices

SNACK
- 10–20 grams of carbohydrates

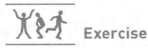 Exercise

REST DAY!

WEEK 3, DAY 6

BREAKFAST
Choose one main dish:
- 2 whole-wheat pancakes, measuring 5 inches across, with 1 tea-spoon of butter and 1 teaspoon of 100 percent maple syrup
- ¾ cup oatmeal or Cream of Wheat, cooked with the option of ¼ cup of nuts (use ground cinnamon for taste if desired)
- 1 cup of cold cereal, not sugar-coated, with ½ cup of skim or reduced-fat milk

Power Ups:
- 1 piece of fruit
- 100% whole-wheat English muffin
- Water (unlimited), 1 cup of tea or 1 cup of black coffee with 1 tablespoon of low-calorie cream or 1 tablespoon of skim or reduced-fat milk, or ½ cup of fresh juice

SNACK
- 10–20 grams of carbohydrates

LUNCH
Choose one main dish:
- 1 slice of cheese pizza and a medium-sized green garden salad with 2 tablespoons of fat-free, light salad dressing
- 1 cup of lentil soup or bean soup and 1 small salad with 2 table-spoons of fat-free, light dressing
- Chicken and Red Pepper Hummus Wraps (recipe page 135)

Power Ups:
- 1 piece of fruit or ½ cup of berries

SNACK
- 10–20 grams of carbohydrates

DINNER
Choose one main dish:
- 5 ounces of skinless, boneless chicken, grilled/baked
- Caesar salad with or without chicken (only ¼ cup of croutons and only 2 tablespoons of fat-free, light salad dressing)
- Easy Shepherd's Pie (recipe page 161)

Power Ups:
- 2 servings of vegetables, if you choose the chicken

SNACK
- 10–20 grams of carbohydrates

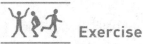 ## Exercise

- 20 minutes: Cardiovascular/aerobic activity in the morning
- 20 minutes: Cardiovascular/aerobic activity in the late afternoon/evening

WEEK 3, DAY 7

BREAKFAST

Choose one main dish:

- 1 cup cold cereal, not sugar-coated, with ½ cup skim or reduced-fat milk
- 12-ounce fruit smoothie (300 calories or less, no sugar or other sweeteners added)
- Egg and Veggie Breakfast Sandwich (recipe page 123)

(recipe page 123)

Power Ups:

- 1 piece of fruit or ½ cup of berries, if you choose the cereal or egg sandwich
- Water (unlimited), 1 cup of tea or 1 cup of black coffee with 1 tablespoon of low-calorie cream, or ½ cup of fresh juice

SNACK

- 10–20 grams of carbohydrates

LUNCH

Choose one main dish:

- ½ cup tuna salad in a 100% whole-grain or 100% whole-wheat pita
- Chicken sandwich on 2 slices of 100% whole-grain or 100% whole-wheat toast with lettuce, tomato, and 1 teaspoon of mayonnaise or mustard
- 1 cup tomato, black bean, lentil, chicken, or vegetable soup

Power Ups:
- Small green garden salad with 1 tablespoon of fat-free, light salad dressing

SNACK
- 10–20 grams of carbohydrates

DINNER
Choose one main dish:
- 1 cup of whole-grain pasta, drizzled with olive oil and garlic, with 4 ounces of meatballs (chicken or turkey)
- 5 ounces of fish, grilled/baked
- 5 ounces of steak, grilled

Power Ups:
- 1 small baked sweet potato
- 1 serving of vegetables
- 1 whole-wheat dinner roll

SNACK
- 10–20 grams of carbohydrates

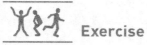 ## Exercise

- 20 minutes: Cardiovascular/aerobic activity
- 20 minutes: Resistance exercises

6 WEEK 4: CHALLENGE

Congrats on making it to week 4! Your body should be adapting to the changes you have made. Your sugar cravings should be reduced, and you are now more satisfied with foods that are full of proper nourishment and great fuel for your body to feel and look better. The body is a wonderful machine, and it is equally stubborn. When you repeatedly introduce it to the same challenges, it no longer responds as dramatically or as consistently as it has in the past. Now it's time to switch course a little.

You will still be eating healthier foods and making smarter choices, but we are going to change your meal types and the order in which you eat them. This week is dedicated to creating a new challenge, one that you certainly can handle, but will take you a little out of your comfort zone. Face this week with a positive attitude and remind yourself that this change in your routine will only increase and enhance the results that you already have achieved. The mind is what leads and the body follows. This week is as much about your mental as it is your physical execution. Focus and most important have fun!

BAD HABIT _____

CHANGE _____

GOOD HABIT _____

IMPROVABLE HABIT _____

CHANGE _____

Here is just a sample of what your daily schedule might look like this week. Remember, your schedule is based on the time you wake up and go to sleep, so you need to fill it in accordingly. This is built for someone who gets up at 7 A.M. If you need an emergency snack after dinner because you're hungry, make sure you choose something that is 5 grams of carbs or less and no more than 150 calories.

Wake Up	Breakfast	Snack	Snack	Snack	Dinner
7 A.M.	8 A.M.	10 A.M.	12:30 P.M.	3:30 P.M.	6:30–7PM

WEEK 4, DAY 1

BREAKFAST

Choose one main dish:

- 1 or 2 scrambled eggs, cooked in oil or cooking spray, salt and pepper to taste
- 1 cup of cold cereal, not sugar-coated, with ½ cup of skim, or reduced-fat milk
- Avocado and Grapefruit Toasts (recipe page 118)

Power Ups:

- ½ cup of fresh strawberries, sliced, or 1 piece of medium-sized fruit

SNACK

- 10–20 grams of carbohydrates

SNACK

- 10–20 grams of carbohydrates

SNACK

- 10–20 grams of carbohydrates

DINNER

Choose one main dish:

- 6 ounces of fish (salmon, halibut, tuna, trout), grilled/baked (NOT fried)
- Roasted Eggplant Rollatini (recipe page 150)

NUTRI NUGGET

Sugars are molecules composed of carbon, hydrogen, and oxygen. The simplest sugars include glucose, fructose, and galactose. Table sugar is the crystal form of sucrose, which is a fusion of one fructose and one glucose molecule.

Power Ups:
- 2 servings of vegetables

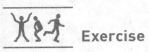 Exercise

- 20 minutes: Cardiovascular/aerobic activity in the morning
- 20 minutes: Cardiovascular/aerobic activity in the late after-noon/evening

WEEK 4, DAY 2

BREAKFAST

Choose one main dish:

- 8-ounce fruit smoothie with no sugar or other sweeteners added
- 1 slice of french toast with 1 teaspoon of 100 percent maple syrup
- Breakfast Grits with Oranges and Pecans (recipe page 120)

Power Ups:

- If you choose the smoothie, you can also have 2 slices of 100% whole-grain or 100% whole-wheat toast with a small amount of butter or sugar-free jelly spread
- If you choose the french toast, you can also have ½ cup of berries

SNACK

- 10–20 grams of carbohydrates

SNACK

- 10–20 grams of carbohydrates

SNACK

- 10–20 grams of carbohydrates

DINNER

Choose one main dish:

- Vegetarian plate of 3 vegetable servings
- 5 ounces of boneless pork chops, grilled/baked, trimmed of fat
- Beef and Pepper Stir-Fry (recipe page 158)

Power Ups:

If you're having the pork chops or beef and pepper stir-fry, you can also have the sides below:

- ½ cup of steamed or grilled cauliflower
- ½ cup of cooked brown rice

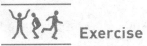 **Exercise**

- 15 minutes: Cardiovascular/aerobic activity
- 20 minutes: Resistance training

WEEK 4, DAY 3

BREAKFAST
Choose one main dish:
- Omelet with diced vegetables
- 1 cup of cold cereal, not sugar-coated, with ½ cup skim, or reduced-fat milk
- Oatmeal with Apples, Almonds, and Cinnamon (recipe page 122)

Power Ups:
- 1 medium apple
- 1 slice of 100% whole-grain or 100% whole-wheat toast with 1 teaspoon butter or sugar-free jelly spread

SNACK
- 10–20 grams of carbohydrates

SNACK
- 10–20 grams of carbohydrates

SNACK
- 10–20 grams of carbohydrates

FIBER: DAILY RECOMMENDATIONS FOR ADULTS

	Age 50 or younger	Age 51 or older
Men	38 grams	30 grams
Women	25 grams	21 grams

Source: Institute of Medicine

DINNER

Choose one main dish:

- 5 ounces of fish, grilled
- Chicken stir-fry (use 6 ounces of chicken, low-sodium soy sauce, and 1 cup of veggies)
- Grilled Lamb Chops with Chickpea and Feta Relish (recipe page 163)

Power Ups:

- 1 cup of vegetables
- ½ cup of cooked brown rice

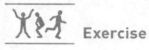 **Exercise**

REST DAY!

WEEK 4, DAY 4

BREAKFAST

Choose one main dish:

- 1 cup of oatmeal or Cream of Wheat with ½ cup of skim or reduced-fat milk
- 1 breakfast burrito (scrambled egg, bell pepper, and onion in a warm, 100% whole-wheat tortilla, sprinkled with 1 tablespoon of salsa and 1 tablespoon of shredded nonfat cheese)
- Egg and Turkey Sausage Mini Breakfast Pizza (recipe page 117)

Power Ups:

- 1 piece of fruit

SNACK

- 10–20 grams of carbohydrates

SNACK

- 10–20 grams of carbohydrates

SNACK

- 10–20 grams of carbohydrates

DINNER

Choose one main dish:

- 6 ounces of chicken breast, grilled/baked with roasted lemon
- 5 ounces of shrimp, grilled/baked

--- NUTRI NUGGET ---

Research shows that fructose, a popular type of sugar, can damage the liver much like alcohol. Fructose is what makes fruit taste so sweet, and in this naturally occurring form it is fine. But when fructose is manipulated, such as in extractions from corn, sugarcane, and beets, it can harm the liver.

Source: Journal of Hepatology; 2013, 58(2), 395–398 and Nature; 2012, 487(5), 27–29.

- Curried Squash, Onion, and Lentil Stew (recipe page 169)

Power Ups:
- 1 cup of vegetables (you can have ½ cup of one vegetable and ½ cup of another)
- ½ cup of cooked brown rice

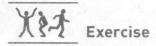 **Exercise**

- 35 minutes: Cardiovascular/aerobic activity

WEEK 4, DAY 5

BREAKFAST

Choose one main dish:

- 1 cup of whole-grain, high-fiber cereal with ½ cup skim or reduced-fat milk
- 6 ounces of nonfat plain yogurt with ¼ cup of granola, ¼ cup of blueberries, and 1 tablespoon of chopped nuts, if desired
- Mini Huevos Rancheros (recipe page 119)

Power Ups:

- 1 cup of berries
- 1 slice of 100% whole-wheat or 100% whole-grain toast with butter and 1 teaspoon sugar-free jelly spread (only if you choose the cereal option)

SNACK

- 10–20 grams of carbohydrates

SNACK

- 10–20 grams of carbohydrates

DINNER

Choose one main dish:

- 5 ounces of chicken, grilled/baked, or 5 ounces of pork chop, grilled/baked
- Large green garden salad with diced chicken and 2 tablespoons of fat-free, light salad dressing

---

NUTRI NUGGET

Sugar addiction is a real and sometimes serious condition. According to a brain scan study from the US National Institute on Drug Abuse, sugar can affect the brain similar to the way cocaine and alcohol impact it. These changes can lead to more cravings for sugar.
Source: Nature Reviews Neuroscience; 2004, 5(12), 963–970. Food and Addiction: A Comprehension Handbook;2012, Oxford University Press

- Turkey Salisbury Steaks with Mushroom Sauce (recipe page 167)

Power Ups:
- 1 medium baked sweet potato
- 1 cup of vegetables

 Exercise

- 35 minutes: Cardiovascular/aerobic activity

WEEK 4, DAY 6

BREAKFAST

Choose one main dish:
- 1 cup of oatmeal or Cream of Wheat with ½ cup of skim or reduced-fat milk
- ½ whole-grain bagel spread with 1 tablespoon of light cream cheese and 1 teaspoon of low-sugar fruit spread
- Egg and Spinach Frittata with Feta (recipe page 124)

Power Ups:
- 1 slice of 100% whole-grain or 100% whole-wheat toast
- ½ cup of berries

SNACK
- 10–20 grams of carbohydrates

SNACK
- 10–20 grams of carbohydrates

SNACK
- 10–20 grams of carbohydrates

DINNER

Choose one main dish:
- Vegetarian plate of 3 servings of vegetables
- 5-ounce slice of meat loaf made from lean beef
- Spicy Green Chile Pork Stew (recipe page 165)

Power Ups:
- ½ cup of cooked brown rice
- ½ cup of green beans

 Exercise

REST DAY!

WEEK 4, DAY 7

BREAKFAST

Choose one main dish:

- 1 croissant with 1 egg, 1 slice of fat-free or reduced-fat cheese, and 1 slice of bacon
- 2 whole-wheat pancakes, measuring 5 inches across, with 1 teaspoon of butter and 1 teaspoon of 100 percent maple syrup
- Roasted Pepper and Scallion Strata (recipe page 121)

SNACK

- 10–20 grams of carbohydrates

SNACK

- 10–20 grams of carbohydrates

SNACK

- 10–20 grams of carbohydrates

DINNER

Choose one main dish:

- Barbecue chicken (4 ounces of chicken tender strips or 2 drumsticks with 2 tablespoons of barbecue sauce)
- 5 ounces of fish, grilled/baked
- Kale Caesar Salad with Poached Chicken (recipe page 131)

> ### — NUTRI NUGGET —
> Snacking can be a great shortcut to a healthy lifestyle. An estimated 70 percent of Americans use snacking as a way to incorporate fruits and vegetables into their diets.
> *Source: Produce for Better Health Foundation*

Power Ups:
- ½ cup of steamed broccoli
- ½ cup of mashed sweet potatoes (use fat-free buttermilk instead of cream, and unsalted butter)

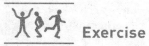 Exercise

- 15 minutes: Cardiovascular/aerobic activity
- 20 minutes: Resistance exercises

7 WEEK 5: BLAST

You've made it to week 5, the final unique week of your transformation. This week combines all that you have learned and tried the last four weeks. The idea behind this week is that you will blast off into a lifestyle that doesn't require a manual for the rest of your life. Now you can make smarter, healthier choices. This program's intention is not to teach you how to be perfect but rather to teach you how to make nutritional decisions that will help you live longer, feel stronger, and provide your body with the nourishment that will help you stave off disease.

Sugar is a universal compound that is found in natural and processed foods. It's virtually unavoidable even with the healthiest of eating behaviors. Our goal is to *reduce* the amount of added sugars and emphasize natural sugars—those that are naturally found in food—and help you choose and create foods that are extremely tasty and satisfying. After this week, you can still follow portions or the entire program or customize it to what will fit your lifestyle. If you find yourself getting off track, pick up at any week and do as much of it as you want. This plan becomes your guide and you make it work for you. Embrace your new way of living and only look back to see how far you've come!

BAD HABIT _____

CHANGE _____

GOOD HABIT _____

IMPROVABLE HABIT _____

CHANGE _____

WEEK 5, DAY 1

BREAKFAST

Choose one main dish:
- 1 or 2 scrambled eggs cooked in olive oil or cooking spray, salt and pepper to taste
- 2 pancakes (4½ inches across) with 1 tablespoon of 100 percent maple syrup
- Oatmeal with Apples, Almonds, and Cinnamon (recipe page 122)

Power Ups:
- 1 piece of fruit
- Water (unlimited), 1 cup of tea or 1 cup of black coffee with 1 tablespoon of low-calorie cream or 1 tablespoon of skim or reduced-fat milk, or ½ cup of fresh juice

SNACK
- 10–20 grams of carbohydrates

LUNCH

Choose one main dish:
- Grilled chicken salad (2 cups of mixed greens with 3 ounces

---

NUTRI NUGGET

Eat:
- **More vegetables,** especially non-starchy ones (no potatoes, corn, or peas). And watch the salt.
- **Whole-grain foods** (think whole-wheat bread) over refined grains and flour. Half the grains you eat should be whole grains.
- **Lean proteins.** Fish at least twice a week, and beans or soy instead of meat, when you can. When you do eat meat, go lean (pork loin or sirloin). And remove the skin from your chicken.
- **Fruit.** Fresh is best. If you choose canned or frozen, make sure it has no added sugar.
- **Fats.** They're OK in small amounts if you're eating healthy fats, like those from avocados, olives, nuts, or seeds. Avoid the full-fat cheeses and full-fat milk. No regular butter or creamy sauces. And put back those potato chips and fatty snacks.

Source: American Diabetes Association

of skinless diced chicken, ⅓ cup of diced bell pepper, ⅓ cup of diced onion, 5 cherry tomatoes, ⅓ cup of shredded carrot, and 2 tablespoons of fat-free, light salad dressing)

- Roast beef sandwich on 100% whole-grain or 100% whole-wheat bread, with 1 teaspoon of mayonnaise or mustard and 1 slice of fat-free or reduced-fat cheese

Power Ups:
- ½ cup of raw vegetables

SNACK
- 10–20 grams of carbohydrates

DINNER
Choose one main dish:
- 5 ounces of fish, grilled
- 1 cup of whole-wheat spaghetti with meat sauce
- Grilled Beef Eye Round Steaks with Red Pepper Relish (recipe page 160)

Power Ups:
- ½ cup of brown rice
- ½ cup of broccoli

SNACK
- Fewer than 10 grams of carbohydrates

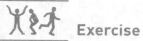 Exercise

- 20 minutes: Cardiovascular/aerobic activity in the morning
- 20 minutes: Cardiovascular/aerobic activity in the late afternoon/evening

WEEK 5, DAY 2

BREAKFAST
Choose one main dish:
- 1 cup of cold cereal, no sugar added, with ½ cup of skim or reduced-fat milk
- 1 croissant with 1 egg, 1 slice of fat-free or reduced-fat cheese, and 1 slice of bacon

Power Ups:
- ½ large grapefruit or 8 melon balls

SNACK
- 10–20 grams of carbohydrates

LUNCH
Choose one main dish:
- 1 whole-wheat tortilla chicken wrap (4 ounces of chicken, 1 teaspoon of hummus, ½ cup of mixed greens, 1 teaspoon of fat-free or reduced-fat cheese, and ¼ cup of sun-dried tomatoes, optional)
- 1 cup of chicken noodle soup
- Tuna Melt Muffins (recipe page 139)

Power Ups:
- ½ cup of vegetables
- 8 small whole-wheat crackers

SNACK
- 10–20 grams of carbohydrates

DINNER

Choose one main dish:

- 1 cup of whole-wheat spaghetti with 4 small 1-inch meatballs in marinara sauce
- 5 ounces of pan-seared steak with herbs
- 5 ounces of skinless, boneless chicken, grilled/baked

Power Ups:

- 1 cup of vegetables divided into 2 types (e.g., ½ cup squash and ½ cup carrots)

SNACK

- Fewer than 10 grams of carbohydrates

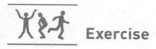 Exercise

- REST DAY!

WEEK 5, DAY 3

BREAKFAST

Choose one main dish:

- 1 yogurt parfait (1 cup of nonfat plain yogurt with ½ cup of fresh fruit)
- Grilled cheese sandwich on 2 slices of 100% whole-grain or 100% whole-wheat bread
- 1 cup of oatmeal with ½ cup skim or reduced-fat milk, ½ teaspoon honey, and 1 teaspoon of butter, optional

Power Ups:

- 1 slice of whole-grain toast with ½ teaspoon of sugar-free jelly spread, if you chose the yogurt or oatmeal
- 1 piece of fruit with all three main dish choices

SNACK

- 10–20 grams of carbohydrates

LUNCH

Choose one main dish:

- Veggie cheeseburger on 100% whole-grain or 100% whole-wheat bun
- Ham and cheese sandwich with 4 ounces of ham on 2 slices of 100% whole-wheat or 100% whole-grain bread, with 1 slice of reduced-fat or fat-free cheese, 1 teaspoon of mayonnaise or mustard
- 1 cup of lentil, mushroom, or tomato soup

Power Ups:

- 1 small apple

- Six ¼-inch-thick cucumber slices with 1 teaspoon of fat-free, light salad dressing for dipping

SNACK
- 10–20 grams of carbohydrates

DINNER
Choose one main dish:
- 5 ounces of fish, grilled/baked
- Vegetarian plate with 3 servings of vegetables
- Grilled Chicken Paillard with Arugula and Shaved Parmesan (recipe page 148)

Power Ups:
- 1 whole-grain roll
- ½ cup of brown rice

SNACK
- Fewer than 10 grams of carbohydrates

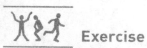 Exercise

- 20 minutes: Cardiovascular/aerobic activity
- 20 minutes: Resistance exercises

WEEK 5, DAY 4

BREAKFAST

Choose one main dish:
- 1 cup of cold cereal, no sugar added, with ½ cup of skim or reduced-fat milk
- 1 cup of hot cooked cereal (such as steel-cut oatmeal, grits, or Cream of Wheat) with ½ cup of skim or reduced-fat milk
- Egg and Veggie Breakfast Sandwich (recipe page 123)

Power Ups:
- ¾ cup of fresh blueberries or sliced strawberries

SNACK
- 10–20 grams of carbohydrates

LUNCH

Choose one main dish:
- Roast beef sandwich (3 ounces of lean roast beef, lettuce, and slice of tomato on 2 slices of 100% whole-grain or 100% whole-wheat bread, with 1 teaspoon of mayonnaise or mustard)
- Tuna melt (1 toasted whole-wheat English muffin topped with ⅓ cup of tuna mixed with 1 tablespoon of mayonnaise, 1 teaspoon of relish, and 1 ounce of fat-free or reduced-fat cheese)
- Chicken salad (2 cups of mixed greens, ¼ cup of sliced red grapes, 3 ounces of cooked chicken breast, 6 slices of cucumbers, and 1 stalk of chopped celery, optional, drizzled with 2 tablespoons of fat-free, light salad dressing)

Power Ups:
- 1 small piece of fruit

SNACK
- 10–20 grams of carbohydrates

DINNER
Choose one main dish:
- 2½ × 4-inch slice of meat lasagna
- Barbecue chicken (4 ounces of chicken tender strips or 2 drumsticks with 2 tablespoons of barbecue sauce)
- Curried Squash, Onion, and Lentil Stew (recipe page 169)

Power Ups:
- 1 cup of steamed or grilled vegetables
- 1 small 100% whole-grain or 100% whole-wheat roll

SNACK
- Fewer than 10 grams of carbohydrates

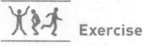 Exercise

- 35 minutes: Cardiovascular/aerobic activity

WEEK 5, DAY 5

BREAKFAST

Choose one main dish:

- 1 fresh peach sliced with ½ cup of low-fat, low-sodium cottage cheese
- 1 egg, scrambled with 1 ounce of fat-free or reduced-fat cheese with olive oil or cooking spray
- 1 cup of cold cereal, no sugar added, with ½ cup of skim or reduced-fat milk

Power Ups:

- 1 small apple, orange, or banana
- 2 slices of 100% whole-grain or whole-wheat bread or 100% whole-grain or whole-wheat English muffin

SNACK

- 10–20 grams of carbohydrates

LUNCH

Choose one main dish:

- Grilled chicken with lettuce and tomato on 100% whole-grain or 100% whole-wheat toast with 1 teaspoon of mayonnaise or mustard
- 1 cup vegetable soup topped with 1 teaspoon of nonfat plain yogurt and 5 halved cherry tomatoes
- Turkey wrap in a whole-wheat pita with 4 ounces of turkey and lettuce, tomato, and low-calorie dressing

Power Ups:
- 1 small green garden salad with 1 tablespoon of fat-free, light salad dressing

SNACK
- 10–20 grams of carbohydrates

DINNER
Choose one main dish:
- 5 ounces of fish, grilled
- Tofu stir-fry (4 ounces of tofu, with 2 cups of mixed veggies cooked in 2 tablespoons of low-sodium stir-fry sauce and 1 tablespoon of olive oil; served over 1 cup of cooked brown rice)
- Caesar salad with or without chicken (only ¼ cup of croutons and only 2 tablespoons of salad dressing)

Power Ups:
- ½ cup of cooked cabbage
- ½ cup of mashed sweet potatoes (use fat-free buttermilk instead of cream, and unsalted butter)

SNACK
- Fewer than 10 grams of carbohydrates

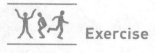 Exercise

- REST DAY!

WEEK 5, DAY 6

BREAKFAST

Choose one main dish:

- 1 cup of hot cooked cereal with ½ cup of skim or reduced-fat milk
- 12-ounce fruit smoothie (250 calories or less and 30 grams carbs or less)
- 1 whole-grain or whole-wheat waffle (5 inches in diameter) with ½ tablespoon of 100 percent maple syrup

Power Ups:

- 2 strips of pork or turkey bacon

SNACK

- 10–20 grams of carbohydrates

LUNCH

Choose one main dish:

- 1 cup of whole-wheat pasta with ¼ cup of tomato sauce and vegetables
- 1 whole-wheat tortilla chicken wrap (4 ounces of chicken, 1 teaspoon of hummus, ½ cup of mixed greens, 1 teaspoon of fat-free or reduced-fat cheese, and ¼ cup sun-dried tomatoes, optional)
- Hearty Minestrone Soup (recipe page 137)

Power Ups:

- 1 cup of brown rice, if you choose the chicken wrap or soup
- 1 small green garden salad with 1 tablespoon of fat-free, light salad dressing

SNACK
- 10–20 grams of carbohydrates

DINNER

Choose one main dish:
- 5 ounces of salmon or other fish, grilled/baked
- 5 ounces of skinless, boneless chicken, grilled/baked
- Vegetarian plate, 3 servings of vegetables

Power Ups:
- 1 cup of cooked brown or wild rice, if you choose any of the main dishes
- 1 cup of steamed summer squash, if you choose the fish or chicken

SNACK
- Fewer than 10 grams of carbohydrates

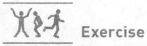 Exercise

- 20 minutes: Cardiovascular/aerobic activity
- 20 minutes: Resistance exercises

WEEK 5, DAY 7

BREAKFAST
Choose one main dish:
- 12-ounce fruit smoothie (250 calories or less and 30 grams carbs or less)
- 1 cup of cold cereal, no sugar added, with ½ cup of skim or reduced-fat milk
- 8-ounce yogurt parfait with granola and fruit
- Egg and Spinach Frittata with Feta (recipe page 124)

Power Ups:
- 1 small piece of fruit

SNACK
- 10–20 grams of carbohydrates

LUNCH
Choose one main dish:
- Turkey wrap in a whole-wheat pita with 4 ounces of turkey and lettuce, tomato, and fat-free, light salad dressing
- Tuna salad sandwich on 100% whole-grain or 100% whole-wheat bread
- Roasted Butternut Squash and Spinach Salad (recipe page 129)

Power Ups:
- ½ cup of berries or 1 small piece of fruit

SNACK
- 10–20 grams of carbohydrates

DINNER

Choose one main dish:

- Pan-seared steak (5 ounces)
- Chicken stir-fry with vegetables (1½ cups)
- 1½ cups of soup (carrot, tomato, lentil, vegetable, chicken, pea)

Power Ups:

- 1 cup of vegetable medley, if you choose the steak
- ½ cup of brown or dirty rice, with all the main dish choices
- 1 whole-grain roll

SNACK

- Fewer than 10 grams of carbohydrates

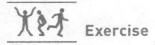 Exercise

- 35 minutes: Cardiovascular/aerobic activity

8 BLAST THE SUGAR OUT SNACKS

Snacking is an extremely important part of any weight loss program, but particularly so for those who are prediabetic or diabetic. Snacks can be a great way to boost your energy between meals, and they can prevent you from feeling too hungry as you wait for your next meal. Snacking wisely is critically important because it will help keep you full while at the same time prevent you from consuming too many calories and spiking your blood sugars, something that you are trying your best to avoid. Snacks that have fiber and lots of nutrients are the best choices to curb your appetite. Although salty or sweet snacks might be your preference occasionally, think of snacks as another opportunity to fit in another serving of whole grains, fruits, or vegetables—low-calorie options that will keep your hunger at bay until your next meal. Remember that portion sizes always make a big difference and can help you keep better control of your blood glucose. Preparation, like most things in life, is to your advantage. If you take a few minutes to plan ahead, you can avoid making bad decisions or finding yourself unable to locate appropriate and beneficial snacks. Below are some snack options that you can select from. Of course, it's impossible to compile a list that encompasses *every* snack possibility, but this is a good start!

SNACKS WITH FEWER THAN 5 GRAMS OF CARBOHYDRATES

- 15 almonds
- 3 celery sticks + 1 tablespoon of peanut butter
- 5 baby carrots
- 5 cherry tomatoes + 1 tablespoon of ranch dressing
- 1 hard-boiled egg
- 1 cup cucumber slices + 1 tablespoon of ranch dressing
- ¼ cup of fresh blueberries
- 1 cup of salad greens + ½ cup of diced cucumber + drizzle of vinegar and oil
- 1 sugar-free popsicle
- 1 cup of air-popped popcorn such as SHRED POP
- 2 saltine crackers
- 10 Goldfish crackers
- ½ cup sugar-free Jell-O
- 1 reduced-fat string cheese stick
- 8 green olives
- 2 tablespoons of pumpkin or sesame seeds
- ¼ of a whole avocado (approximately 4 grams)
- Ants on a Log: Celery sticks (3) spread with peanut butter (⅓ tablespoon on each) and topped with 2 raisins (6 total)
- Cream Cheese and Cucumber Chipwiches: Cucumber sliced into "chips" (1 cup), with each "chip" spread with light cream cheese (3 tablespoons total) and topped with another cucumber "chip." Sprinkle with some dried dill for a flavor kick!
- Ham/Turkey and Cheese Roll-Ups: Thinly sliced deli meats spread with mustard, layered with a thinly sliced piece of cheese, and rolled up

- Lettuce Wraps: Large leaf of lettuce (the greener the lettuce the better!) filled with either tuna, chicken, or egg salad (½ cup) and eaten like a taco
- Veggie Dunkers: Raw veggie sticks (mixture of carrot, cucumber, pepper, zucchini, yellow squash, celery, broccoli, cauliflower—½ cup) dipped in fat-free, light salad dressing, salsa, or guacamole (2 tablespoons)
- Spinach Pepper Boats: Scooped and seeded bell pepper sliced in half, stuffed with premade spinach dip, and sprinkled with parmesan cheese (½ medium bell pepper, 3 tablespoons dip)
- Peanut (or other nut) butter: Approximately 1 tablespoon
- Almonds, Brazil nuts, peanuts, pecans, macadamia nuts, walnuts: Lightly salted or unsalted, approximately ¼ cup (approximately 1 ounce)
- Cashews, pistachios, soy nuts: Lightly salted or unsalted, approximately ⅛ cup (approximately 0.5 ounce)
- Sunflower seeds/pumpkin seeds: Lightly salted or unsalted, approximately ⅛ cup (approximately 0.5 ounce)
- Avocado: ⅓ cup sliced/chunks
- Edamame (green soybeans): ¼ cup of shelled
- Tuna, chicken, or egg salad: ½ cup
- Sugar-free Jell-O and 1 tablespoon of whipped cream
- ½ cup diced fruit plus 2 tablespoons of low-sugar whipped topping
- String cheese (made with 2 percent milk): 1 stick
- Sugar-free popsicles: 1 popsicle
- Hard-boiled egg (1 egg) or 2 halves of deviled eggs

SNACKS WITH ABOUT 10–20 GRAMS OF CARBOHYDRATES

- ¼ cup of dried fruit and nut mix
- 1 cup of chicken noodle soup, tomato soup (made with water), or vegetable soup
- 1 small apple or orange
- 3 cups of air-popped popcorn such as SHRED POP
- ⅓ cup of hummus + 1 cup of raw, sliced veggies (bell pepper, carrots, broccoli, cucumber, celery, cauliflower, or a combination of these)
- ¼ cup of cottage cheese + ½ cup of canned or fresh fruit
- 1 cheese quesadilla (made with one 6-inch corn or whole-wheat tortilla + 1 ounce of shredded cheese) + ¼ cup of salsa
- Two 4-inch rice cakes + 1 tablespoon of peanut butter
- 5 whole-wheat crackers (or ¾ ounce) + 1 piece of string cheese
- ½ turkey sandwich (1 slice of whole-wheat bread + 2 ounces of turkey + mustard)
- ½ cup of tuna salad + 4 saltine crackers
- ¾ cup of unsweetened dry cereal
- ½ cup of cooked cereal
- ½ of 6-inch pita
- ¼ of a large whole-grain bagel
- 2 Stella D'Oro breadsticks
- ½ of an English muffin
- 2 Wasa crackers
- One 4-inch 100% whole-grain or 100% whole-wheat waffle or pancake (4 inches across)
- 2 large rice cakes
- 6 saltine crackers

- 7 Ritz crackers
- 60 small oyster crackers
- 40 Goldfish crackers
- 4 Melba toast
- 5 Triscuits
- 12 Wheat Thins
- 1 small granola bar (about 15-gram carb size)
- 2–5 whole-wheat crackers
- 8 animal crackers
- 6 vanilla wafers
- 3 graham crackers (2 ½-inch square)
- 3 gingersnaps
- 100-calorie packs (crackers and cookies)
- 3 peanut-butter sandwich crackers
- 3 cups air-popped popcorn
- 6 tablespoons of hummus
- 2 pretzel rods
- 10 pretzel nibblers
- ¾ ounces pretzels
- ½ soft pretzel
- 10 baked potato chips
- 11 baked Doritos
- 10–15 snack chips (baked potato, pita, or tortilla chips)
- ½ cup ice cream or frozen yogurt
- ½ cup of no-sugar-added ice cream
- 1 frozen fruit juice bar
- ½ cup of sugar-free pudding
- 1 ounce of trail mix
- 1 cup of milk (8 ounces)
- 6 ounces of low-fat or fat-free yogurt

- 1 cup of soy milk (8 ounces)
- 1 small apple, orange, pear
- 1 medium peach or nectarine
- 2 small clementine oranges
- 12 Bing cherries
- ½ banana
- 2 small plums
- 1 kiwi
- 3 prunes
- 2 tablespoons of dried fruit
- ½ grapefruit
- 17 small grapes or 8 large grapes
- 1 cup of berries
- 1½ cups cubed/balls of watermelon
- 4 pineapple rings
- 1 cup or ⅓ of melon, cantaloupe, or honeydew
- ½ cup of light or packed-in-own juice canned fruit (strain the juice)
- ½ cup of juice (orange, grapefruit, apple, cranberry juice cocktail, or cider)
- ⅓ cup of grape or prune juice

ABOUT 30 GRAMS OF CARBOHYDRATES (GOOD TO EAT BEFORE EXERCISE)

- ½ peanut butter sandwich (1 slice of 100% whole-grain or 100% whole-wheat bread with 1 tablespoon of peanut butter)
- 1¾ cup of berries (blueberries, blackberries, raspberries, or

a combination of these) with 1 cup of milk or 6 ounces of light yogurt

- 1 English muffin + 1 teaspoon of low-fat margarine
- ¾ cup whole-grain, ready-to-eat cereal + ½ cup of skim milk
- 1 medium banana + 1 tablespoon of peanut butter

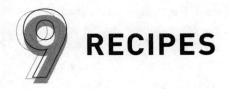 **RECIPES**

BREAKFAST RECIPES

TOMATO-ASPARAGUS BREAKFAST CASSEROLE

EGG AND TURKEY SAUSAGE MINI BREAKFAST PIZZAS

AVOCADO AND GRAPEFRUIT TOASTS

MINI HUEVOS RANCHEROS

BREAKFAST GRITS WITH ORANGES AND PECANS

ROASTED PEPPER AND SCALLION STRATA

OATMEAL WITH APPLES, ALMONDS, AND CINNAMON

EGG AND VEGGIE BREAKFAST SANDWICH

EGG AND SPINACH FRITTATA WITH FETA

SMOKED SALMON WRAP WITH CAPERS, RED ONION, AND ARUGULA

TOMATO-ASPARAGUS BREAKFAST CASSEROLE

SERVES 4

Nutritional Information Per Serving: 232 cal., 12 g fat, 5 g sat. fat, 16 g carb., 16 g protein, 339 mg sodium, 3 g sugar, 6 g fiber

½ small bunch asparagus, about 4 ounces, trimmed and cut into 1-inch pieces

2 100% whole-grain or 100% whole-wheat English muffins, split and roughly chopped into small pieces

2 vine-ripened tomatoes, thinly sliced

4 large eggs

½ cup reduced-fat milk

2 tablespoons finely grated parmesan cheese

⅛ teaspoon salt

¼ teaspoon freshly ground black pepper

¼ teaspoon dried basil or parsley

½ cup shredded low-fat mozzarella cheese

1. Preheat the oven to 330 degrees F.

2. Bring a small saucepan filled with water to a boil. Drop the asparagus into the water and cook for 2 minutes, then drain. Scatter the muffin pieces into the bottom of an 8-inch square baking pan. Scatter the asparagus over the muffin pieces and lay the tomato slices over the top, slightly overlapping. In a medium bowl, whisk the eggs, milk, parmesan, salt, pepper, and basil together until combined. Pour the mixture over the muffins and vegetables in the pan and let stand for 10 minutes until the liquid is absorbed. Scatter the mozzarella over the top and bake in the oven until set and the cheese is melted and beginning to brown, 15 to 20 minutes.

3. Let stand 10 minutes before cutting and serving warm or at room temperature.

EGG AND TURKEY SAUSAGE MINI BREAKFAST PIZZAS

SERVES 4

Nutritional Information Per Serving: 191 cal., 8 g fat, 3 g sat. fat, 14 g carb., 15 g protein, 415 mg sodium, 2 g sugar, 2 g fiber

Cooking spray
2 fully cooked low-sodium turkey sausage breakfast patties, finely chopped
3 large eggs
¼ teaspoon dried Italian seasoning
¼ teaspoon salt
Pinch freshly ground black pepper
½ cup jarred low-sugar marinara sauce
2 100% whole-grain or 100% whole-wheat English muffins, split and toasted
¼ cup shredded low-fat mozzarella

1. Position an oven rack 6 inches from the broiler and preheat the broiler on medium or low.

2. Spray a medium nonstick skillet with cooking spray and heat it over medium heat. Add the turkey sausage and cook, stirring frequently, until crisp, 6 to 8 minutes. Reduce the heat to low. Meanwhile, in a bowl whisk together the eggs, Italian seasoning, salt, and pepper until combined. Pour the eggs into the pan and, using a rubber spatula, cook them slowly, stirring, until just set. Remove from the heat.

3. Spread 2 tablespoons of the marinara sauce on each of the muffin halves, put one-quarter of the cooked eggs on each muffin half and top with some shredded mozzarella. Broil until the sauce is bubbling and cheese is melted, about 5 minutes. Serve warm.

AVOCADO AND GRAPEFRUIT TOASTS

SERVES 4

1 ripe avocado, peeled, pitted, and
    thinly sliced
4 slices 100% whole-grain or sprouted
    grain bread, toasted
Pinch salt
Freshly ground black pepper, to taste
1 ruby red grapefruit
½ teaspoon honey

Nutritional Information Per Serving: 187 cal., 7 g fat, 1 g sat. fat, 27 g carb., 5 g protein, 143 mg sodium, 9 g sugar, 6 g fiber

1. Arrange one quarter of the sliced avocado on each toast slice and season lightly with salt and pepper.

2. Using a sharp knife, cut the peel and pith away from the grapefruit membrane. Hold the fruit in one hand and carefully cut the segments away from the membrane, dropping them into a bowl. Squeeze the membrane to extract any juice left in it. Divide the grapefruit segments among the avocado-topped toast slices; reserve the juice for later or drink it with your breakfast.

3. Drizzle a little honey over each toast slice and serve.

MINI HUEVOS RANCHEROS

SERVES 4

4 no-salt-added corn tortillas (6 inches in diameter)

Cooking spray

1 can (16-ounce) low-fat, low-sodium refried beans

4 large eggs

¼ teaspoon salt

Freshly ground black pepper, to taste

1½ ounces grated Monterey Jack cheese

½ cup fresh tomato salsa

1 avocado, diced

Hot sauce, for serving

Nutritional Information Per Serving: 359 cal., 15 g fat, 5 g sat. fat, 35 g carb., 19 g protein, 470 mg sodium, 3 g sugar, 9 g fiber

1. Preheat the oven to 375 degrees F.

2. Warm the tortillas in the microwave or oven. Spray one side of the tortillas lightly with cooking spray and tuck them, oiled side down, into the compartments of a jumbo muffin tin, creating bowls.

3. Fill each tortilla cup with one quarter of the refried beans and spread it evenly into the bottom of the tortilla. Crack an egg into each cup and season the eggs with salt and pepper. Bake until the eggs are set and the tortilla cups are beginning to crisp, 10 to 12 minutes. Remove the pan from the oven, evenly sprinkle the cheese over the tops of the eggs, and return the pan to the oven for 2 to 3 minutes to melt the cheese.

4. To serve, put the tortilla-egg cups into four small bowls. Garnish with salsa and diced avocado and serve warm with hot sauce on the side.

BREAKFAST GRITS WITH ORANGES AND PECANS

SERVES 4

1½ cups nonfat milk or low-fat soy or
   almond milk
½ cup instant grits
1 teaspoon honey
Finely grated zest of 1 lemon
⅛ teaspoon ground ginger
4 ounces no-sugar-added canned
   mandarin oranges, drained
¼ cup chopped pecans, toasted

Nutritional Information Per Serving: 208 cal., 5 g fat, 0 g sat. fat, 19 g carb., 6 g protein, 68 mg sodium, 12 g sugar, 3 g fiber

1. Bring the milk to a simmer in a medium saucepan over medium heat. Gradually whisk the grits into the liquid, reduce the heat to low, and simmer until thickened. Stir in the honey, lemon zest, and ginger.

2. Divide the grits among 4 warm bowls, top each with some orange segments and pecans and serve.

ROASTED PEPPER AND SCALLION STRATA

SERVES 4

Nutritional Information Per Serving: 175 cal., 7 g fat, 3 g sat. fat, 15 g carb., 11 g protein, 251 mg sodium, 4 g sugar, 4 g fiber

2 slices 100% whole-grain or sprouted bread, toasted and cut into small cubes

1 jarred roasted red bell pepper, drained and chopped

6 scallions, sliced

Cooking spray

4 large eggs

½ cup low-fat milk

2 tablespoons finely grated parmesan cheese

1 tablespoon Dijon mustard

¼ teaspoon freshly ground black pepper

¼ teaspoon smoked paprika

⅛ teaspoon garlic powder

1. Preheat the oven to 350 degrees F.

2. In a small bowl, toss together the bread cubes, bell peppers, and scallions until combined. Spray one 8×5-inch nonstick loaf pan lightly with cooking spray, and spread the bread mixture evenly in the pan.

3. In a medium bowl, whisk together the eggs, milk, parmesan, mustard, black pepper, paprika, and garlic powder until combined. Pour the egg mixture over the bread mixture in the pan and press the bread down into the liquid with a rubber spatula. Let stand for about 15 minutes until the bread absorbs the liquid.

4. Bake the strata until the bread is set and beginning to puff and turn golden, 20 to 25 minutes.

5. Cool in the pan for about 5 minutes before slicing and serving warm.

OATMEAL WITH APPLES, ALMONDS, AND CINNAMON

SERVES 4

Nutritional Information Per Serving: 218 cal., 7 g fat, 1 g sat. fat, 35 g carb., 6 g protein, 8 mg sodium, 6 g sugar, 6 g fiber

1 teaspoon butter
1 Honeycrisp or Gala apple, peeled and diced
½ teaspoon ground cinnamon
3½ cups water
2 cups old-fashioned oats
¼ cup sliced almonds, toasted

1. Melt the butter in a medium saucepan over medium heat and add the apples and cinnamon. Cook, stirring, until apples soften slightly, about 5 minutes. Transfer the apples to a bowl.

2. Add the water to the pan and bring to a boil over medium-high heat. Stir in the oats and cooked apples, reduce the heat to a simmer, and cook, stirring frequently, until oats are soft but not mushy, 3 to 4 minutes.

3. Divide the oatmeal among 4 bowls, top each with almonds and serve.

EGG AND VEGGIE BREAKFAST SANDWICH

MAKES 4

Nutritional Information Per Serving: 202 cal., 6 g fat, 2 g sat. fat, 30 g carb., 17 g protein, 344 mg sodium, 2 g sugar, 9 g fiber

Cooking spray
3 large egg whites
1 large egg
⅛ teaspoon salt
⅛ teaspoon freshly ground black pepper
4 100% whole-grain English muffins, split and toasted
½ jar roasted red bell peppers, sliced into thin strips
½ cup quartered artichoke hearts in water, drained and coarsely chopped
¾ cup shredded low-fat mozzarella

1. Spray a nonstick medium skillet with cooking spray and heat over medium-low heat.

2. In a small bowl, whisk the egg whites and whole egg, salt, and black pepper together until combined. Pour the eggs into the skillet and, using a rubber spatula, stir gently until the eggs are cooked but still soft, 2 to 3 minutes.

3. Set the muffin bottoms on each of 4 plates. Divide the red pepper strips and chopped artichokes among the muffins. Spoon a quarter of the cooked eggs onto each muffin and sprinkle some cheese over each. Top each with the muffin top and serve immediately.

EGG AND SPINACH FRITTATA WITH FETA

SERVES 4

Nutritional Information Per Serving: 109 cal., 6 g fat, 3 g sat. fat, 3 g carb., 11 g protein, 362 mg sodium, 1 g sugar, 1 g fiber

4 large egg whites
2 large eggs
⅛ teaspoon salt
Pinch freshly ground black pepper
Pinch freshly grated nutmeg
Pinch cayenne pepper
Cooking spray
1 cup frozen spinach, thawed and squeezed dry
2 ounces feta cheese, finely crumbled
1 tablespoon finely grated parmesan cheese

1. Preheat the oven to 375° F.

2. In a medium bowl, whisk the egg whites, eggs, salt, pepper, nutmeg, and cayenne together until combined.

3. Spray an oven-proof medium nonstick skillet generously with cooking spray and heat over medium-low heat. Pour in the egg mixture and let stand for about 1 minute, until the eggs begin to set around the edges. Using a rubber spatula, pull a little of the eggs around the edge into the center, letting the liquid egg run into the edges.

4. Scatter the spinach and feta evenly over the eggs, sprinkle the parmesan over the top. Transfer the pan to the oven and bake until the egg is completely set on top and beginning to brown, 5 to 8 minutes.

5. Carefully remove the pan from the oven and run a rubber spatula under the frittata to release it. Slide it onto a serving plate, cut into four pieces, and serve warm.

SMOKED SALMON WRAP WITH CAPERS, RED ONION, AND ARUGULA

SERVES 4

Nutritional Information Per Serving: 103 cal., 4 g fat, 2 g sat. fat, 15 g carb., 8 g protein, 305 mg sodium, 4 g sugar, 2 g fiber

2 large (12-inch) no-salt-added 100% whole-wheat tortillas
¼ cup low-fat cream cheese
¼ cup nonfat yogurt
Freshly ground black pepper, to taste
2 ounces smoked salmon, coarsely chopped
1 tablespoon capers in brine, drained
¼ small red onion, very thinly sliced
1 cup fresh arugula or baby spinach leaves

1. Lay the tortillas on a work surface. In a small bowl, beat the cream cheese with a rubber spatula, fork, or wooden spoon until softened. Add the yogurt and whip until combined. Divide the cream cheese mixture between the tortillas and spread it evenly over the surface of each tortilla, grind black pepper over each.

2. Scatter the salmon, capers, onion, and greens over the surface of the tortillas. Working one at a time, fold two sides of the tortilla over about 2 inches, and then roll the tortilla up tightly like a burrito. Repeat with the second wrap then slice each wrap evenly into two pieces and serve.

LUNCH RECIPES

MEXICAN GRILLED SHRIMP SALAD

ROASTED BUTTERNUT SQUASH AND SPINACH SALAD

KALE CAESAR SALAD WITH POACHED CHICKEN

CURRY CHICKEN SKEWERS

CHICKEN AND RED PEPPER HUMMUS WRAPS

CAULIFLOWER SOUP WITH TOASTED PEPITAS

HEARTY MINESTRONE SOUP

CARROT GINGER SOUP WITH LEMON YOGURT SWIRL

TUNA MELT MUFFINS

TURKEY WALDORF SALAD

CURRIED TURKEY LETTUCE WRAPS

PESTO CHICKEN SALAD SANDWICH

QUICK TURKEY–WHITE BEAN CHILI

MEXICAN QUINOA CHICKEN SALAD

TURKEY-QUINOA BURGERS

CLASSIC CUCUMBER GAZPACHO

MEXICAN GRILLED SHRIMP SALAD

SERVES 4

Nutritional Information Per Serving: 55 cal., 1 g fat, 0 g sat. fat, 5 g carb., 6 g protein, 206 mg sodium, 2 g sugar, 1 g fiber

12 large shrimp, peeled and deveined
2 teaspoons fresh lime juice
1 teaspoon vegetable oil
½ teaspoon chili powder
Pinch garlic powder
salt and freshly ground black pepper, to taste
¼ cup nonfat plain yogurt
⅛ teaspoon ground cumin
2 cups arugula leaves, mixed greens, or baby spinach leaves
1 large tomato, sliced
Lime wedges, for serving

1. On a work surface, slice the shrimp in half horizontally. In a medium bowl, whisk together the lime juice, oil, chili powder, and garlic powder until combined. Add the shrimp, season with the salt and pepper, and toss well to combine. Marinate for at least 10 minutes and no more than 30.

2. Heat a stovetop grill pan over medium-high heat. Working in batches, if necessary, grill the shrimp, turning once, until grill marks appear and the shrimp are bright pink and translucent, about 2 minutes per side. Transfer the shrimp to a clean bowl and let stand until cool.

3. Add the yogurt and cumin to the shrimp and toss well to coat. To serve, divide the greens among 4 plates and top the greens with a couple of tomato slices. Nestle the shrimp salad on top of the tomatoes on each plate and serve with lime wedges on the side for squeezing.

ROASTED BUTTERNUT SQUASH AND SPINACH SALAD

SERVES 4

Nutritional Information Per Serving: 140 cal., 7 g fat, 1 g sat. fat, 19 g carb., 3 g protein, 169 mg sodium, 5 g sugar, 3 g fiber

2 cups peeled and seeded butternut squash cubes, about 1 inch in diameter

1 large shallot, sliced

2 teaspoons olive oil

¼ teaspoon ground cinnamon

¼ teaspoon ground cardamom

Salt and freshly ground black pepper, to taste

½ cup apple juice

4 cups baby spinach leaves

¼ cup chopped pecans, toasted

1. Preheat the oven to 350 degrees F.

2. Put the squash cubes and shallot into a medium bowl. In another small bowl, stir together the oil, cinnamon, and cardamom, and drizzle it over the vegetables. Toss well to coat. Season the squash lightly with salt and pepper and scatter the vegetables in a single, even layer on a baking sheet. Roast in the oven, turning several times with a spatula, until the squash is fork-tender and the shallot has begun to brown and crisp, 20 to 25 minutes.

3. Meanwhile, put the apple juice into a small saucepan and bring to a simmer over medium-low heat. Cook until the liquid has reduced to about 2 tablespoons and is thick and syrupy, 5 to 8 minutes.

4. Put the spinach into a large mixing bowl. When the squash is cooked and still hot, add it to the bowl with the spinach. Pour the reduced apple juice over the salad, season lightly with salt and pepper, and toss until well combined and the spinach begins to wilt.

5. Divide among 4 bowls, top each with pecans and serve.

KALE CAESAR SALAD WITH POACHED CHICKEN

SERVES 4

Nutritional Information Per Serving: 279 cal., 10 g fat, 2 g sat. fat, 13 g carb., 34 g protein, 266 mg sodium, 1 g sugar, 4 g fiber

1 clove garlic, smashed
Juice of 1 lemon, divided
¼ teaspoon whole black peppercorns
1 bay leaf
2 skinless, boneless chicken breasts, about 6 ounces each
2 tablespoons olive oil
½ teaspoon Dijon mustard
Freshly ground black pepper, to taste
1 small bunch kale, about 12 ounces, stemmed and leaves chopped into one-inch pieces
¼ cup finely grated parmesan cheese, plus more for garnish

1. Fill a medium saucepan with 2 inches of water and add the garlic clove, half of the lemon juice, peppercorns, and bay leaf, and bring to a simmer over medium-low heat. Gently slide the chicken breasts into the pan, being sure they are completely submerged. Cover and cook, making sure the water is just barely simmering, until the chicken is cooked through, about 10 minutes. Transfer the chicken to a plate and let stand until cool enough to handle. Using two forks, shred the chicken into bite-sized pieces.

2. Meanwhile, in a small bowl, whisk the oil, mustard, and remaining lemon juice together until thick and emulsified, season with a little black pepper. Put the kale into a large mixing bowl. Pour the dressing over the kale in a mixing bowl and, using tongs,

toss until the leaves are well coated in dressing. Add the parmesan and toss well to combine.

3. To serve, divide the kale among 4 serving plates and evenly scatter the shredded chicken over the salad. Garnish with a sprinkling of parmesan and some fresh black pepper.

CURRY CHICKEN SKEWERS

SERVES 4

¼ cup nonfat plain yogurt

Juice of 1 lime, plus wedges
for serving

½ teaspoon honey

1 teaspoon curry powder

Pinch cayenne pepper

¼ teaspoon salt

1 pound unbreaded chicken tenders

Cooking spray

Steamed brown rice or green salad,
for serving

Nutritional Information Per Serving: 187 cal., 1 g fat, 0 g sat. fat, 20 g carb., 24 g protein, 336 mg sodium, 8 g sugar, 1 g fiber

1. In a small bowl, whisk the yogurt, lime juice, honey, curry, pepper, and salt together until combined. Add the chicken tenders and toss to coat. Let stand for about 15 minutes.

2. Meanwhile, soak about 1 dozen bamboo skewers (for as many chicken tenders that you have) in water for about 10 minutes. Carefully thread the marinated chicken onto the skewers, piercing it every ½ inch.

3. Preheat a stovetop grill pan over medium-high heat.

4. Spray the chicken on both sides with cooking spray and place them on the pan with the exposed skewers hanging over the edge and not in direct contact with the pan. Cook, turning once, until the chicken is cooked through and beginning to brown, 2 to 3 minutes per side. (The skewers can also be broiled, but be sure to cover the exposed skewer ends with aluminum foil to prevent them from burning).

5. Serve the skewers over rice or a green salad, garnished with lime wedges.

CHICKEN AND RED PEPPER HUMMUS WRAPS

SERVES 4

Nutritional Information Per Serving: 353 cal., 9 g fat, 2 g sat. fat, 23 g carb., 50 g protein, 346 mg sodium, 4 g sugar, 6 g fiber

¼ cup store-bought plain hummus
1 piece (about 1×3 inches) jarred roasted red pepper, drained
Pinch smoked paprika
2 large (12-inch) no-salt-added 100% whole-wheat tortillas or wraps
2 cups shredded hormone-free rotisserie chicken, skin removed
2 stalks celery, very thinly sliced lengthwise
4 scallions, thinly sliced

1. Put the hummus, red pepper, and paprika into a small food processor and pureé until combined. Place the tortillas on a work surface and spread half of the hummus over the surface of each. Scatter half of the chicken over the hummus on each tortilla. Position half of the celery horizontally over the lower third of each tortilla and scatter the sliced scallions over the chicken. Working one tortilla at a time, fold the outer edges of the tortilla over the ends of the celery stalks and roll the tortilla up like a burrito. Repeat with the second wrap.

2. Slice each wrap in half crosswise and serve half a wrap per person.

CAULIFLOWER SOUP WITH TOASTED PEPITAS

MAKES ABOUT 1½ QUARTS
SERVES 4 TO 6

Nutritional Information Per Serving: 88 cal., 4 g fat, 1 g sat. fat, 13 g carb., 5 g protein, 306 mg sodium, 3 g sugar, 2 g fiber

1 teaspoon olive oil
½ small white onion, chopped
1 stalk celery, diced
3 cloves garlic, smashed
1 small head cauliflower, stem removed and cut into florets
1 small russet potato, about 6 ounces, peeled and diced
¾ quart low-sodium nonfat chicken stock
1 bay leaf
¼ teaspoon salt, plus more as needed
Freshly ground black pepper
Freshly squeezed lemon juice, to taste
¼ cup toasted pepitas (baby pumpkin seeds)

1. Heat the oil in a large saucepan over medium heat. Add the onion, celery, and garlic. Cook, stirring, until softened, 4 to 5 minutes. Add the cauliflower, potato, chicken or vegetable stock, bay leaf, salt, and black pepper and bring to a boil. Reduce the heat to a simmer, cover, and cook until the cauliflower and potato are very soft and falling apart, 25 to 30 minutes. Remove the bay leaf and discard.

2. Working in small batches, transfer the contents of the pan to a blender and pureé until smooth, or use a stick blender to pureé the soup in the pan. Taste the soup and add lemon juice to brighten the flavor and more salt and pepper, if needed.

3. Serve in warm bowls garnished with pepitas.

HEARTY MINESTRONE SOUP

MAKES ABOUT 1½ QUARTS
SERVES 4

1 tablespoon olive oil
1 small yellow onion, diced
2 cloves garlic, minced
1 bay leaf
1 small sprig fresh rosemary, or
    ½ teaspoon dried
1 sprig fresh thyme, or 1 teaspoon dried
¾ of one 28-ounce can low-sodium,
    no-sugar-added diced tomatoes,
    with their juice
1½ cups low-sodium, nonfat chicken
    stock or vegetable broth
¾ of one 16-ounce can low-sodium
    chickpeas, drained and rinsed
1 stalk celery, sliced
¾ of one 16-ounce can low-sodium
    white beans, drained and rinsed
1 cup cooked ditalini pasta or baby
    shells, optional
Freshly ground black pepper, to taste
Finely grated parmesan cheese, for
    serving

Nutritional Information Per Serving: 228 cal., 5 g fat, 1 g sat. fat, 59 g carb., 15 g protein, 405 mg sodium, 3 g sugar, 13 g fiber

1. Heat the oil in a medium saucepan over medium heat. Add the onion, garlic, bay leaf, rosemary, and thyme. Cook, stirring frequently, until softened, about 5 minutes.

2. Add the tomatoes, chicken stock or vegetable broth, and chickpeas and bring to a boil. Reduce the heat to medium-low, cover, and cook until the tomatoes are breaking down, about 20 minutes.

3. Stir in the celery and white beans and simmer for an additional 5 minutes. Remove the bay leaf and add the pasta, if using, and some black pepper. Serve warm with parmesan cheese sprinkled over the top.

CARROT GINGER SOUP WITH LEMON YOGURT SWIRL

MAKES ABOUT 2 QUARTS
SERVES 6

Nutritional Information Per Serving: 73 cal., 3 g fat, 0 g sat. fat, 9 g carb., 3 g protein, 315 mg sodium, 5 g sugar, 2 g fiber

1 tablespoon olive oil
1 medium yellow onion, chopped
1 large garlic clove, smashed
2 tablespoons (about 3-inch piece) fresh ginger, peeled and minced
6 medium carrots, peeled and coarsely chopped
¾ quart low-sodium, nonfat chicken stock or vegetable broth
¼ teaspoon salt
¼ cup low-fat plain yogurt
1 teaspoon fresh lemon juice
Pinch ground cumin
Freshly ground black pepper, to taste

1. Heat the oil in a medium saucepan over medium heat. Add the onion, garlic, and ginger. Cook, stirring, until softened. Add the carrots, chicken stock or vegetable broth, and salt and bring to a boil. Reduce the heat to a simmer, cover, and cook until the carrots are very soft and falling apart, about 40 minutes.

2. Working in small batches, pureé the soup in a blender or use a stick blender to pureé the soup in the pan. In a small bowl, stir together the yogurt, lemon juice, and cumin.

3. To serve, ladle the soup into warm bowls and drizzle about a tablespoon of the yogurt mixture over the top. Garnish with freshly ground black pepper.

TUNA MELT MUFFINS

SERVES 4

1 can (12-ounce) solid white tuna in
  water, drained
2 stalks celery, finely diced
3 scallions, minced
1 small carrot, peeled and finely diced
3 tablespoons nonfat plain yogurt
¼ teaspoon celery seed
Freshly ground black pepper, to taste
2 low-fat 100% whole-wheat English
  muffins, split and toasted
4 slices reduced-fat medium sharp
  cheddar cheese

Nutritional Information Per Serving: 87 cal., 5 g fat, 3 g sat. fat, 17 g carb., 12 g protein, 246 mg sodium, 2 g sugar, 5 g fiber

1. Preheat the broiler.

2. In a medium bowl, stir the tuna, celery, scallions, carrots, yogurt, celery seed, and pepper together until well combined. Spread one quarter of the mixture onto each muffin half and top with a slice of cheese.

3. Place the muffins on a broiler pan and broil until the cheese is melted and bubbly. Serve warm.

TURKEY WALDORF SALAD

SERVES 4

12 ounces turkey cutlets
¼ teaspoon salt
Freshly ground black pepper, to taste
Cooking spray
½ cup water
2 stalks celery, sliced
1 cup red seedless grapes, halved
¼ cup chopped walnuts, toasted
2 tablespoons chopped fresh parsley
4 scallions, sliced
1 tablespoon low-fat mayonnaise
3 tablespoons plain nonfat yogurt
1 teaspoon honey
4 leaves bib lettuce, for serving

Nutritional Information Per Serving: 272 cal., 6 g fat, 1 g sat. fat, 23 g carb., 29 g protein, 302 mg sodium, 20 g sugar, 2 g fiber

1. Season the turkey cutlets with the salt and pepper. Spray a medium nonstick skillet with cooking spray and heat over medium heat. Add the turkey and cook until browned, 3 to 4 minutes. Flip the turkey and cook until the underside is golden, about 3 minutes more. Pour in the water, reduce the heat to medium-low, cover the pan, and cook until the turkey is completely cooked through, 6 to 8 minutes more. Remove the turkey from the skillet and let stand until cool.

2. In a medium bowl, toss the celery, grapes, walnuts, parsley, and scallions together until combined. In a small bowl, whisk together the mayonnaise, yogurt, and honey. Using two forks, shred the turkey cutlets and add them to the bowl with the celery and grapes, add the dressing and toss until well coated and thoroughly mixed.

3. To serve, divide the turkey salad among the lettuce leaves and season with some fresh black pepper.

CURRIED TURKEY LETTUCE WRAPS

SERVES 4

Nutritional Information Per Serving: 346 cal., 4 g fat, 0 g sat. fat, 12 g carb., 58 g protein, 386 mg sodium, 7 g sugar, 2 g fiber

2 cups water
1 garlic clove, smashed
1 bay leaf
½ teaspoon whole black peppercorns
Juice of ½ lemon
1 pound turkey cutlets
½ cup nonfat Greek yogurt
1 teaspoon mild curry powder
¼ teaspoon salt
Freshly ground black pepper, to taste
¼ cup golden raisins
¼ cup sliced almonds, toasted
8 slices vine-ripened tomato
4 large butter or green leaf lettuce leaves

1. Fill a small skillet with 2 cups of water. Add the garlic, bay leaf, peppercorns, and lemon juice and bring the liquid to a simmer over medium heat. Carefully slip the turkey cutlets into the liquid, being sure they are submerged. Reduce the heat to medium low, cover the pan, and simmer gently until the turkey is cooked through, about 10 minutes. Remove the turkey from the pan and let stand until cool enough to handle.

2. Using two forks, shred the turkey meat and put it in a medium bowl. Add the yogurt, curry, salt, pepper, raisins, and almonds and stir until well combined. To assemble the wraps, place 2 slices of tomato into each lettuce leaf and divide the turkey salad among the leaves. Loosely wrap the lettuce around the turkey and serve.

PESTO CHICKEN SALAD SANDWICH

SERVES 4

Nutritional Information Per Serving: 468 cal., 19 g fat, 3 g sat. fat, 41 g carb., 54 g protein, 417 mg sodium, 9 g sugar, 7 g fiber

⅓ cup low-fat mayonnaise

¼ cup prepared pesto sauce

8 slices 100% whole-grain bread or 100% whole-wheat bread, toasted

1½ cups shredded hormone-free rotisserie chicken meat, skin removed

1 celery stalk, finely diced

2 tablespoons finely minced white onion

4 green leaf lettuce leaves

8 slices vine-ripened tomato

Freshly ground black pepper, to taste

1. In a small bowl, stir the mayonnaise and pesto together until combined. Spread a very thin layer of the mixture on top of each slice of bread. Put the chicken into a small bowl along with the celery and onion and add the remaining pesto mayonnaise to the bowl and stir well to combine.

2. To make the sandwiches, place a lettuce leaf on 4 mayonnaise-covered bread slices and put one-quarter of the chicken salad on top of the lettuce. Position 2 slices of the tomato on top of each sandwich and season them lightly with pepper. Place the remaining bread slices on top, cut the sandwiches in half diagonally, and serve.

QUICK TURKEY– WHITE BEAN CHILI

SERVES 4

Nutritional Information Per Serving: 295 cal., 12 g fat, 3 g sat. fat, 28 g carb., 30 g protein, 342 mg sodium, 5 g sugar, 9 g fiber

1 pound lean ground turkey
1 tablespoon olive oil
1 small yellow onion, finely diced
1 small green pepper, stemmed, seeded, and finely diced
2 garlic cloves, minced
2 teaspoons chili powder
¼ teaspoon salt
½ teaspoon black pepper
1 teaspoon tomato paste
1 bay leaf
¾ of one 28-ounce can diced tomatoes, with their juice
1 can (15-ounce) tomato sauce
¾ of one 15-ounce can low-sodium white beans, drained and rinsed
Hot sauce, for serving

1. Heat the oil in a large saucepan over medium heat. Add the turkey and cook, breaking it up with a spoon, until no longer pink and beginning to brown, about 6 minutes. Add the onion, pepper, and garlic. Cook, stirring frequently, until softened, about 5 minutes. Add the chili powder, salt, pepper, and tomato paste and stir until the paste begins to caramelize in the bottom of the pan, 2 to 3 minutes. Add the bay leaf, diced tomatoes and juice, and tomato sauce and stir well. Bring the mixture to a boil, reduce the heat to medium-low, cover, and simmer for about 15 minutes until thickened.

2. Add the white beans and cook until warmed through. Serve with hot sauce at the table.

MEXICAN QUINOA CHICKEN SALAD

SERVES 4

Nutritional Information Per Serving: 383 cal., 14 g fat, 2 g sat. fat, 27 g carb., 24 g protein, 322 mg sodium, 3 g sugar, 4 g fiber

1½ cups diced hormone-free rotisserie chicken meat, skin removed

2 cups cooked quinoa

¾ of one 15-ounce can fire-roasted tomatoes, drained

4 scallions, thinly sliced

2 tablespoons chopped fresh cilantro leaves

2 tablespoons olive oil

1 tablespoon fresh lime juice

½ teaspoon chili powder

¼ teaspoon salt

½ teaspoon dried oregano

¼ teaspoon ground cumin

¼ teaspoon garlic powder

¼ teaspoon freshly ground black pepper

1. Put the chicken, quinoa, tomatoes, scallions, and cilantro leaves into a medium bowl and toss well to combine. In a small bowl, whisk together the oil, lime juice, chili powder, salt, oregano, cumin, garlic powder, and pepper until combined. Pour the dressing over the salad and toss well to coat.

2. The salad can be served immediately or refrigerated for up to 1 day.

TURKEY-QUINOA BURGERS

SERVES 4

1 pound lean ground turkey
½ cup cooked quinoa
1 medium carrot, finely shredded
1 large shallot, minced
2 large eggs
½ teaspoon Dijon mustard
1 teaspoon dried thyme
1 teaspoon Worcestershire sauce
¼ teaspoon salt
¼ teaspoon freshly ground black
   pepper
Cooking spray

Nutritional Information Per Serving: 258 cal., 11 g fat, 4 g sat. fat, 9 g carb., 26 g protein, 325 mg sodium, 2 g sugar, 2 g fiber

1. Put the turkey, quinoa, carrot, and shallot in a medium bowl and mix to combine. In another bowl, whisk the eggs, mustard, thyme, Worcestershire sauce, salt, and pepper together until combined. Add the egg mixture to the turkey and, using your hands, mix until thoroughly combined. Form the mixture into 4 patties about ½-inch thick.

2. Spray a large nonstick skillet with cooking spray and heat over medium heat. Add the burgers and cook until golden brown on the underside, about 5 minutes. Flip the burgers and continue cooking until golden and the patties are completely cooked through, about 5 minutes more. Cool for 5 minutes before serving.

CLASSIC CUCUMBER GAZPACHO

SERVINGS: 4

1 cucumber, peeled and chopped

1 small red bell pepper, stemmed, seeded, and chopped

2 scallions, green parts only, chopped

1 small clove garlic, smashed

½ cup fat-free or low-fat Greek yogurt

1 cup almond milk

1 teaspoon white vinegar

Juice of ½ lemon

Salt and freshly ground black pepper, to taste

Chopped fresh mint, for garnish

Nutritional Information Per Serving: 32 cal., 1 g fat, 0 g sat. fat, 4 g carb., 2 g protein, 255 mg sodium, 2 g sugar, 1 g fiber

1. Combine the cucumber, bell pepper, scallions, garlic, yogurt, buttermilk, vinegar, and lemon juice in a blender and blend until liquefied.

2. Season with salt and pepper to taste. If the soup is too thick, thin with cold water.

3. Serve cold, garnished with mint.

DINNER RECIPES

GRILLED CHICKEN PAILLARD WITH ARUGULA
AND SHAVED PARMESAN

ROASTED EGGPLANT ROLLATINI

BARLEY, QUINOA, AND MUSHROOM-STUFFED PEPPERS

GREEK LAMB MEATBALLS WITH TZATZIKI

GRILLED ASIAN FLANK STEAK WITH STEAMED BOK CHOY

BEEF AND PEPPER STIR-FRY

GARLIC-HERB MARINATED LONDON BROIL

GRILLED BEEF EYE ROUND STEAKS WITH RED PEPPER RELISH

EASY SHEPHERD'S PIE

GRILLED LAMB CHOPS WITH CHICKPEA AND FETA RELISH

SPICY GREEN CHILE PORK STEW

TURKEY SALISBURY STEAKS WITH MUSHROOM SAUCE

CURRIED SQUASH, ONION, AND LENTIL STEW

MEXICAN CAULIFLOWER, CORN, AND PINTO BEAN STEW

PARCHMENT-BAKED SALMON FILLETS WITH FENNEL
AND CHICKPEAS

GOLDEN CARROT SOUP

HEARTY VEGETABLE STEW

GRILLED CHICKEN PAILLARD WITH ARUGULA AND SHAVED PARMESAN

2 skinless, boneless chicken breasts (about 6 ounces each)
1 tablespoon olive oil
Juice of 1 lemon, divided
¼ teaspoon salt
Freshly ground black pepper, to taste
4 cups baby arugula leaves
1 small vine-ripened tomato, seeded and diced
Lemon Pepper Seasoning, to taste
1½-ounce piece parmesan cheese

SERVES 4

Nutritional Information Per Serving: 253 cal., 9 g fat, 3 g sat. fat, 3 g carb., 33 g protein, 343 mg sodium, 1 g sugar, 0 g fiber

1. Using a sharp knife, halve the chicken breasts horizontally. Working one piece at a time, put a chicken breast piece inside a large food storage bag and, using a meat mallet or the back of a heavy pan, pound the chicken to an even ⅛-inch thickness throughout. Repeat with the remaining chicken.

2. Put the chicken in a shallow dish and drizzle the oil and half of the lemon juice over the top, season the chicken with the salt and pepper, and toss the chicken with a pair of tongs to coat with lemon juice and oil. Let stand for 10 minutes.

3. Preheat a stove-top grill pan or gas grill to medium.

4. Grill the chicken, turning once, until grill marks appear and the chicken is cooked through, 2 to 3 minutes per side. Divide the chicken among 4 plates.

5. Put the arugula in a medium bowl along with the tomato. Drizzle the remaining lemon juice over the greens, sprinkle a little lemon pepper seasoning over the top, and toss well to coat. Arrange ¼ of the greens and tomato directly on top of each chicken breast. Using a vegetable peeler, shave thin strips of parmesan over the top of each plate and serve.

ROASTED EGGPLANT ROLLATINI

SERVES 4

Nutritional Information Per Serving: 173 cal., 11 g fat, 1 g sat. fat, 13 g carb., 7 g protein, 325 mg sodium, 7 g sugar, 6 g fiber

2 small globe eggplants
Cooking spray
¼ teaspoon salt
½ teaspoon garlic powder
¼ teaspoon freshly ground black pepper
3 ounces crumbled feta cheese
1 tablespoon extra-virgin olive oil
1 teaspoon Italian seasoning
Pinch red chili flakes, optional
Finely grated zest of 1 lemon
4 cups fresh baby arugula leaves
Balsamic vinegar, as needed
2 tablespoons shredded parmesan cheese

1. Preheat the oven to 400° F.

2. Spray a nonstick baking sheet lightly with cooking spray.

3. Using a sharp knife, cut each eggplant lengthwise into four ½-inch-thick slices. (You may get more than 4 slices out of each eggplant, depending on their size; you will need 8 slices total.) In a small bowl, stir together the salt, pepper, and garlic powder. Lay the eggplant slices on the baking sheet and spray them lightly with cooking spray. Evenly sprinkle the salt mixture over the top surface of the eggplant. Roast in the oven, turning once, until the eggplant slices are very soft but still hold their shape and are beginning to brown, about 20 minutes. Remove from the oven and let stand for 10 minutes.

4.   Meanwhile, in a medium bowl, stir together the feta, oil, Italian seasoning, chili flakes, and lemon zest until combined. Put ⅛ of the cheese mixture on the wide end of each eggplant slice and roll them up tightly into a cigar shape (the eggplant peel will be on the outside edges of the roll. Once all of the eggplant have been rolled up, return the pan to the oven and bake for about 5 minutes, until the cheese has softened.

5.   To serve, divide the arugula among 4 serving plates and put 2 eggplant rolls on each plate. Drizzle some balsamic vinegar over the greens and rolls and sprinkle some shredded parmesan over each plate. Serve warm.

BARLEY, QUINOA, AND MUSHROOM-STUFFED PEPPERS

SERVES 4

Nutritional Information Per Serving: 321 cal., 10 g fat, 4 g sat. fat, 46 g carb., 14 g protein, 361 mg sodium, 8 g sugar, 7 g fiber

4 medium red bell peppers
1 tablespoon extra-virgin olive oil
1 medium yellow onion, chopped
2 garlic cloves, minced
4 ounces cremini (baby bella) mushrooms, sliced
1 cup low-sodium vegetable broth
1 tablespoon Worcestershire sauce
2 cups rinsed and cooked pearl barley
1 cup cooked quinoa
4 ounces low-fat jack cheese, finely diced
4 scallions, thinly sliced
1 tablespoon chopped fresh thyme leaves
¼ teaspoon salt
½ teaspoon freshly ground black pepper

1. Preheat the oven to 375 degrees F.

2. Slice the top ½-inch of each pepper off, remove the seeds, and stand them upright in a shallow baking dish.

3. Heat the oil in a large skillet over medium-high heat. Add the onion and cook, stirring often, until it begins to brown and caramelize, 8 to 10 minutes. Add the garlic, stir, and cook for 1 to 2 minutes. Add the mushrooms and cook, stirring frequently, until the mushrooms are softened, have given off their moisture, and are beginning to brown, about 10 minutes. Add the broth and Worcestershire sauce and cook until the liquid is simmering and reduces slightly. Remove the pan from the heat and stir in the barley and quinoa. Let stand for a few minutes to cool.

4. Stir three-quarters of the cheese, scallions, thyme, salt, and black pepper into the barley mixture and stir well to combine. Divide the barley among the 4 red pepper cups in the baking dish. Top the peppers with the remaining diced cheese, then bake until the peppers are soft when pierced with a knife but still hold their shape, about 20 minutes. Cool for 10 minutes before serving.

GREEK LAMB MEATBALLS WITH TZATZIKI

SERVES 4

Nutritional Information Per Serving: 386 cal., 30 g fat, 14 g sat. fat, 4 g carb., 23 g protein, 328 mg sodium, 1 g sugar, 1 g fiber

For the meatballs:
1 pound ground lamb
1 large shallot, minced
1 large egg
½ teaspoon salt
1 teaspoon dried oregano
1 teaspoon dried mint
½ teaspoon garlic powder
½ teaspoon ground cumin
½ teaspoon freshly ground black
    pepper
½ teaspoon ground coriander
⅓ cup finely crumbled feta cheese

For the tzatziki:
½ English cucumber, peeled
⅓ cup nonfat Greek yogurt
1 tablespoon minced fresh mint or
    1 teaspoon dried
⅛ teaspoon salt
¼ teaspoon freshly ground black
    pepper
¼ teaspoon garlic powder

1. Preheat the oven to 375 degrees F.

2. Line a baking sheet with parchment paper.

3. To make the meatballs, put the lamb in a medium bowl. Add the shallot. In a small bowl, whisk the egg, salt, oregano, mint, garlic powder, cumin, pepper, and coriander together until well combined. Pour the mixture over the lamb and shallot and, using your hands, mix the meat and seasonings together until combined. Add the feta and mix well. Shape the mixture into 12 equal-sized meatballs and place them on the baking sheet. Bake the meatballs

until they begin to brown and are cooked through, 25 to 30 minutes. Cool for 5 minutes before serving.

4. Meanwhile, to make the tzatziki, grate the cucumber on the large holes of a box grater into a bowl. Transfer the grated cucumber to a fine mesh strainer set over another bowl and let drain for about 10 minutes. Press on the cucumber to remove as much moisture as possible and put it into a bowl. Add the yogurt, mint, salt, pepper, and garlic powder and stir well to combine.

5. Serve 3 meatballs per serving with about ⅓ cup of the tzatziki on the side.

GRILLED ASIAN FLANK STEAK WITH STEAMED BOK CHOY

SERVES 4

Nutritional Information Per Serving: 434 cal., 15 g fat, 5 g sat. fat, 24 g carb., 56 g protein, 316 mg sodium, 8 g sugar, 16 g fiber

1-pound flank steak
1 tablespoon vegetable oil
1 tablespoon toasted sesame oil
1 tablespoon rice vinegar
2 teaspoons fresh lime juice
1 teaspoon low-sodium soy sauce
1 clove garlic, minced
1 teaspoon fresh ginger, peeled and minced
Pinch red pepper flakes
Cooking spray
8 heads baby bok choy

1. Put the steak in a shallow dish. In a small bowl, whisk together the oil, sesame oil, vinegar, lime juice, soy sauce, garlic, ginger, and red pepper flakes until combined. Pour the marinade over the meat, toss to coat, and let stand for 15 minutes.

2. Heat a stovetop grill pan over medium-high heat. Remove the steak from the marinade, letting the excess drip off. Spray both sides of the meat lightly with cooking spray. Put the steak on the grill pan and cook until grill marks appear and the meat releases itself from the pan, 4 to 5 minutes. Flip and continue cooking until grill marks appear and the meat is cooked to desired doneness, about 3 to 4 minutes more for medium. Remove the steak from the grill, cover, and let stand for 10 minutes before slicing.

3. Meanwhile, fill a pan with a steamer insert one-third full of water and bring to a boil over high heat. Add the bok choy, cover, and steam until bright green and crisp-tender, 2 to 3 minutes.

4. To serve, put 2 heads of bok choy on each of 4 serving plates. Thinly slice the steak against the grain and divide among the serving plates. Serve warm.

BEEF AND PEPPER STIR-FRY

SERVES 4

Nutritional Information Per Serving: 349 cal., 8 g fat, 1 g sat. fat, 19 g carb., 33 g protein, 87 mg sodium, 3 g sugar, 2 g fiber

12-ounce top round steak, very thinly sliced

1 tablespoon cornstarch, divided

2 tablespoons vegetable oil

1 medium yellow onion, thinly sliced

1 green bell pepper, stemmed, seeded, and thinly sliced

1 red bell pepper, stemmed, seeded, and thinly sliced

2 cloves garlic, minced

1 teaspoon fresh ginger, peeled and finely minced

1 tablespoon low-sodium soy sauce

1 tablespoon rice vinegar

Pinch red pepper flakes, optional

2 cups steamed brown rice, for serving

1. Sprinkle half of the cornstarch over the steak and toss it to coat as evenly as possible. Heat the oil in a wok or large nonstick skillet over medium-high heat until smoking. Add the steak in a single layer and stir-fry until browned and cooked through, 5 to 6 minutes. Transfer the steak to a plate and cover to keep warm.

2. Add the onion and bell peppers to the pan and stir-fry, stirring constantly, until the vegetables have softened, about 5 minutes. Add the garlic and ginger and stir-fry for 1 minute. In a small bowl, whisk the soy sauce, vinegar, red pepper flakes, and remaining cornstarch together. Pour it into the pan, return the steak to the pan, and cook, stirring, until the meat is hot and everything is glazed, 2 to 3 minutes.

3. Divide the stir-fry among 4 serving plates and serve with steamed rice on the side.

GARLIC-HERB MARINATED LONDON BROIL

SERVES 4

Nutritional Information Per Serving: 241 cal., 10 g fat, 1 g sat. fat, 1 g carb., 34 g protein, 219 mg sodium, 0 g sugar, 0 g fiber

1 London broil (top round beef steak, about 1½ pounds)
1 tablespoon extra-virgin olive oil
1 tablespoon red wine vinegar
3 garlic cloves, minced
2 tablespoons chopped fresh parsley
1 tablespoon chopped fresh thyme leaves
1 tablespoon chopped fresh oregano
Cooking spray
¼ teaspoon salt
¼ teaspoon freshly ground black pepper

1. Put the steak in a shallow dish. In a small bowl, whisk together the oil, vinegar, garlic, parsley, thyme, salt, pepper, and oregano. Pour the marinade over the steak and toss to coat. Let stand at room temperature, turning occasionally in the marinade, for 15 to 20 minutes.

2. Arrange an oven rack 4 inches from the heating element and preheat the broiler. Spray the broiler pan with cooking spray. Remove the steak from the marinade and transfer it to the broiler pan. Broil the steak until the top begins to brown, about 4 minutes. Carefully flip the steak and continue broiling until the meat is browning on the surface and cooked to desired doneness, about 4 to 5 minutes more for medium.

3. Remove the steak from the broiler pan, cover it with aluminum foil, and let stand for 10 minutes. Thinly slice the steak against the grain with a sharp knife and serve.

GRILLED BEEF EYE ROUND STEAKS WITH RED PEPPER RELISH

SERVES 4

Nutritional Information Per Serving: 433 cal., 15 g fat, 3 g sat. fat, 8 g carb., 63 g protein, 360 mg sodium, 6 g sugar, 1 g fiber

2 tablespoons olive oil

4 beef eye round steaks, about ½-inch thick (5–7 ounces each)

½ teaspoon salt

Freshly ground black pepper, to taste

1 large shallot, minced

2 garlic cloves, minced

1 red bell pepper, stemmed, seeded, and finely diced

¼ cup red wine vinegar

1 tablespoon honey

1. Heat the oil in a large nonstick skillet over medium-high heat. Season the steaks on both sides with the salt and pepper. Place the steaks in the skillet and cook until seared and browned on the underside, 2 to 3 minutes. Flip the steaks and continue cooking until browned, 2 to 3 minutes more for medium. Transfer the steaks to a plate and cover tightly with aluminum foil to keep warm.

2. Add the shallot and garlic to the pan and cook, stirring, until softened slightly, about 2 minutes. Add the red pepper, vinegar, and honey, reduce the heat to medium-low, and simmer until the pepper is soft and the liquid has evaporated, about 10 minutes.

3. Serve the steaks warm with the hot relish spooned over the top.

EASY SHEPHERD'S PIE

SERVES 4

Nutritional Information Per Serving: 308 cal., 13 g fat, 5 g sat. fat, 19 g carb., 27 g protein, 376 mg sodium, 6 g sugar, 3 g fiber

2 large Yukon Gold potatoes (about 12 ounces), peeled and diced
3 tablespoons nonfat Greek yogurt
½ teaspoon salt, divided
1 tablespoon olive oil
12 ounces lean ground beef
1 small yellow onion, chopped
1 tablespoon all-purpose flour
¾ of one 15-ounce can low-sodium beef broth
1 tablespoon Worcestershire sauce
1 cup frozen diced carrots
1 cup frozen pearl onions
4 scallions, sliced, green parts only

1. Put the potatoes in a medium saucepan, cover with water, and bring to a boil over medium-high heat. Cook until very soft, 10 to 12 minutes, drain and transfer to a medium bowl. Add the yogurt and ¼ teaspoon of the salt and mash with a potato masher until smooth. Set aside while you make the filling.

2. Preheat the broiler.

3. Heat the oil in a large nonstick skillet over medium-high heat and add the beef. Cook, breaking it up with a wooden spoon, until browned and beginning to crisp, about 10 minutes. Add the yellow onion and cook, stirring, until softened, 2 to 3 minutes. Sprinkle the flour over the beef, stir well, and cook for 1 or 2 minutes. Add the beef broth, Worcestershire sauce, carrots, pearl onions, and remaining salt and bring the mixture to a simmer.

Cook until the liquid has thickened and the vegetables are heated through, about 5 minutes. Stir in the scallions.

4. Transfer the beef filling to an ovenproof 1-quart baking dish. Spoon the mashed potatoes over the top of the filling, spreading it evenly to completely cover the filling. Place the dish under the broiler and broil until the potatoes begin to brown and the filling is bubbling around the edges, about 5 minutes.

5. Let stand for 10 minutes before serving.

GRILLED LAMB CHOPS WITH CHICKPEA AND FETA RELISH

SERVES 4

Nutritional Information Per Serving: 409 cal., 43 g fat, 18 g sat. fat, 30 g carb., 73 g protein, 384 mg sodium, 10 g sugar, 5 g fiber

8 small lamb chops from a rack, about 5 ounces each
1 tablespoon extra-virgin olive oil
1 teaspoon fresh lemon juice
¼ teaspoon dried thyme
¼ teaspoon dried rosemary
¼ teaspoon salt
¼ teaspoon freshly ground black pepper
½ of one 15-ounce can low-sodium chickpeas, drained, rinsed, and coarsely chopped
1 small shallot, minced
1 teaspoon red wine vinegar
¼ teaspoon honey or agave syrup
¼ teaspoon dried oregano
1½ ounces crumbled feta

1. Put the lamb chops in a shallow dish. In a small bowl, whisk the oil, lemon juice, thyme, rosemary, salt, and pepper together until combined. Pour the marinade over the lamb and toss them to evenly coat in the marinade. Let stand for at least 10 minutes.

2. Meanwhile, put the chickpeas and shallot into a mixing bowl and toss to combine. Whisk together the vinegar, honey, and oregano, and pour it over the chickpeas. Add the feta and toss lightly until just combined.

3. Preheat a grill pan over medium-high heat until very hot and nearly smoking.

4. Grill the lamb chops until grill marks appear, 2 to 3 minutes.

Flip the lamb chops and continue grilling until browned on the underside, 2 to 3 minutes more for medium.

5. Serve the lamb chops warm with the chickpea relish spooned over the top.

SPICY GREEN CHILE PORK STEW

SERVES 4

Nutritional Information Per Serving: 400 cal., 24 g fat, 7 g sat. fat, 38 g carb., 34 g protein, 325 mg sodium, 2 g sugar, 4 g fiber

2 tablespoons vegetable oil

1½ pounds pork shoulder, trimmed well and cut into 1½-inch cubes

2 tablespoons all-purpose flour

1 medium yellow onion, chopped

2 cloves garlic, minced

3 cups low-sodium chicken stock

2 poblano chiles

2 medium jalapeño chiles

1 small bunch cilantro

Juice of 1 lime

½ teaspoon salt

¼ teaspoon freshly ground black pepper

2 cups cooked brown rice, for serving

1. Heat the oil in a large saucepan over medium-high heat. Toss the pork cubes in the flour until coated and add half of the pork cubes to the pan and cook, turning often, until browned, about 5 minutes. Transfer the pork to a plate and brown the remaining pork in the pan. Remove the browned pork and add the onion to the pan. Cook, stirring, until softened, about 5 minutes. Add the garlic and cook for 1 or 2 minutes more. Return the browned pork to the pan, along with any accumulated juices, add the stock and cook, scraping up any browned bits on the bottom of the pan, until the liquid begins to boil. Cover the pan, lower the heat to medium-low, and simmer until the pork is tender, about 30 minutes.

2. Meanwhile, preheat the broiler. Put the poblanos and jalapeños on a baking sheet and put the pan under the broiler. Cook until the peppers begin to blacken, 6 to 8 minutes. Turn the peppers and

continue broiling until they are blackened and soft, about 5 minutes more. Transfer the peppers to a bowl, cover the bowl with plastic wrap, and let stand for 5 minutes.

3. Remove the peppers from the bowl and use a paper towel to rub the blackened skins from them. Cut the stems, seeds, and ribs away from the peppers and transfer the flesh to a food processor. Add the cilantro, stems and all, to the processor and pulse the mixture until coarsely ground.

4. After the pork has cooked for 30 minutes, add the pureéd pepper mixture to the pan and stir well. Add the lime juice, salt, and black pepper, and bring the mixture to a simmer. Continue cooking until the pork is fork-tender, 15 to 20 minutes more.

5. Serve the stew hot in bowls with a scoop of rice on the side.

TURKEY SALISBURY STEAKS WITH MUSHROOM SAUCE

SERVES 4

Nutritional Information Per Serving: 309 cal., 18 g fat, 5 g sat. fat, 6 g carb., 28 g protein, 395 mg sodium, 2 g sugar, 0 g fiber

2 tablespoons olive oil, divided

1 small yellow onion, finely chopped

1 clove garlic, minced

3 tablespoons Worcestershire sauce, divided

1 pound lean ground turkey

½ teaspoon salt

½ teaspoon freshly ground black pepper

½ teaspoon dried thyme

½ teaspoon dried parsley

2 large eggs, beaten

4 ounces cremini (baby bella) mushrooms, sliced

1 teaspoon low-sodium soy sauce

¾ of one 15-ounce can low-sodium beef broth

2 tablespoons nonfat Greek yogurt

1. Heat 1 tablespoon of the oil in a large nonstick skillet over medium heat. Add the onion and garlic and cook, stirring, until softened, about 5 minutes. Add 1 tablespoon of the Worcestershire sauce and cook until it begins to bubble. Remove from the heat and pour the onion mixture into a medium mixing bowl, cool to room temperature.

2. Add the turkey, salt, pepper, thyme, and parsley to the cooled onion. Using your hands, mix well until combined. Whisk the second tablespoon of Worcestershire sauce and eggs together and add it to the turkey. Mix well with your hands and divide the mixture into 4 equal portions. Shape each portion into an oval, about ½-inch thick.

3. Add the remaining oil to the skillet that the onion was cooked in and heat over medium-high heat. Add the turkey patties and cook until golden brown on the underside, about 5 minutes. Flip the patties, reduce the heat to medium-low, cover the pan, and continue cooking until completely cooked through and golden brown, 6 to 8 minutes more. Transfer the steaks to a plate and cover with aluminum foil to keep warm.

4. Return the pan to the stove over medium-high heat. Add the mushrooms and cook, stirring, until they release their liquid and begin to brown, 6 to 8 minutes. Add the third tablespoon of Worcestershire sauce, soy sauce, and broth and bring the mixture to a boil. Cook until the liquid has reduced by about half, about 5 minutes. Remove from the heat and stir in the yogurt.

5. Serve the Salisbury steaks warm with the hot mushroom sauce spooned over the top.

CURRIED SQUASH, ONION, AND LENTIL STEW

SERVES 4

Nutritional Information Per Serving: 382 cal., 4 g fat, 0 g sat. fat, 89 g carb., 7 g protein, 32 mg sodium, 32 g sugar, 14 g fiber

1 small butternut squash (about 1 pound), peeled, seeded, and cut into 1-inch pieces
1 tablespoon vegetable oil
1 medium yellow onion, chopped
3 cloves garlic, minced
1 teaspoon tomato paste
1 teaspoon honey
½ teaspoon salt
½ teaspoon turmeric
½ teaspoon mild curry powder
1 small bay leaf
Pinch red pepper flakes
2 cups vegetable broth
2 cups cooked red lentils
¼ cup chopped fresh cilantro
3 scallions, sliced
¼ cup nonfat Greek Yogurt

1. Preheat the oven to 375 degrees F.

2. Line a baking sheet with parchment paper and spread the squash in an even layer on the pan. Roast the squash in the oven until easily pierced with a knife, about 15 minutes.

3. Meanwhile, heat the oil in a large saucepan over medium heat. Add the onion and garlic and cook, stirring, until softened, about 5 minutes. Add the tomato paste, honey, and salt. Cook, stirring, until the tomato paste begins to caramelize, 2 to 3 minutes. Add the turmeric, curry powder, bay leaf, and pepper flakes, and stir for about 1 minute to toast the spices. Pour in the broth and stir well, when it begins to simmer, add the roasted squash and cook until the liquid reduces slightly and thickens, about 5 minutes.

4. Stir in the lentils and cilantro and cook until bubbling again. Remove from the heat.

5. Divide the stew among 4 deep bowls. Sprinkle the scallions over the top and garnish each bowl with a tablespoon of yogurt. Serve hot.

MEXICAN CAULIFLOWER, CORN, AND PINTO BEAN STEW

SERVES 4

Nutritional Information Per Serving: 268 cal., 5 g fat, 0 g sat. fat, 47 g carb., 10 g protein, 315 mg sodium, 8 g sugar, 12 g fiber

1 small head cauliflower, cored and cut into bite-sized florets
1 tablespoon vegetable oil
1 medium yellow onion, chopped
1 small jalapeño chile, stemmed, seeded, ribs removed, and minced
1 clove garlic, minced
½ teaspoon ground cumin
½ teaspoon chili powder
¼ teaspoon salt
3 tablespoons all-purpose flour
2 cups low-sodium vegetable broth
1 cup frozen corn kernels
1 can (15-ounce) pinto beans, drained
Juice of 1 lime
3 tablespoons chopped fresh cilantro, leaves only
4 small (6-inch) no salt added 100% whole-wheat tortillas, warmed, for serving

1. Preheat the oven to 400 degrees F.

2. Line a baking sheet with parchment paper and scatter the cauliflower evenly over the pan. Bake in the oven until the edges turn golden brown and crispy, about 15 minutes. Remove from the oven.

3. Heat the oil in a large saucepan over medium-high heat. Add the onion, jalapeño, and garlic. Cook, stirring, until softened, about 5 minutes. Add the cumin, chili powder, and salt, and stir for about 1 minute. Sprinkle the flour over the vegetables, stir well, and cook for 2 to 3 minutes. Whisk in the broth and bring the mixture to a boil. Reduce the heat and simmer until the liquid has thickened,

about 5 minutes. Add the corn and cook, stirring frequently, until the liquid returns to a boil.

4. Stir in the beans and roasted cauliflower and simmer until the stew is very hot. Remove from the heat and stir in the lime juice.

5. Divide the stew among 4 large bowls and sprinkle some cilantro over each. Fold the tortillas into quarters and serve on the side for dipping.

PARCHMENT-BAKED SALMON FILLETS WITH FENNEL AND CHICKPEAS

SERVES 4

Nutritional Information Per Serving: 402 cal., 26 g fat, 6 g sat. fat, 26 g carb., 45 g protein, 305 mg sodium, 1 g sugar, 8 g fiber

1 small bulb fennel, trimmed, cored, and fronds reserved

1 can (14-ounce) low-sodium chickpeas, drained and rinsed

½ teaspoon dried basil

½ teaspoon dried dill

1 tablespoon cold unsalted butter, cut into small cubes

4 center-cut skinless salmon fillets, preferably wild (6-ounces each)

¼ teaspoon salt

Freshly ground black pepper, to taste

1 lemon, very thinly sliced and seeds removed

1. Preheat the oven to 400 degrees F.

2. Using a mandolin slicer or very sharp knife, slice the fennel into paper-thin slices crosswise and put them in a bowl. Add the chickpeas, basil, and dill, toss to combine.

3. Arrange 4 large sheets of parchment paper (about 12 inches long) on a work surface. Divide the fennel mixture among the parchment sheets, arranging in a flat, single layer on the center of each sheet. Dot each pile of fennel with some butter cubes. Place a salmon fillet directly on top of the fennel on each parchment sheet. Sprinkle the salt and pepper evenly over the fish and lay 2 or 3 lemon slices on top.

4. Bring the ends of each parchment sheet together and fold them tightly down over the top of the salmon, fold up the ends and tuck them under the salmon to enclose the salmon and vegetables completely. Transfer the packets to a baking sheet. Bake until the salmon is cooked through, about 20 minutes.

5. To serve, put a packet on each of four plates and open them at the table. Chop the fennel fronds and sprinkle them over the top of the salmon to garnish.

GOLDEN CARROT SOUP

SERVINGS: 4

1 cup chopped onion
½ teaspoon minced garlic
2 tablespoons butter
2 cups sliced carrots
4 cups water
¼ cup brown rice
4 teaspoons chicken bouillon
½ cup of skim or reduced-fat milk
4 tablespoons minced fresh parsley

Nutritional Information Per Serving: 160 cal., 6 g fat, 4 g sat. fat, 23 g carb., 3 g protein, 94 mg sodium, 5 g sugar, 3 g fiber

1. In a medium saucepan, sauté onion and garlic in butter until tender. Add the carrots, and toss until coated with butter. Add rice, water, and bouillon and bring to a boil. Reduce heat, cover, and simmer for 20 to 25 minutes or until carrots and rice are very tender.

2. Remove from the heat, cool slightly. Transfer to a blender or food processor one-third at a time and blend until smooth. Return to the saucepan, add milk, and heat through. Sprinkle with parsley and serve.

HEARTY VEGETABLE STEW

SERVINGS: 4

Nutritional Information Per Serving: 207 cal., 10 g fat, 2 g sat. fat, 21 g carb., 7 g protein, 281 mg sodium, 7 g sugar, 6 g fiber

2 cups water, hot
1 large yellow onion, chopped
1 clove garlic, minced
8 ounces button mushrooms
One 10-ounce package frozen peas
1 cup chopped celery
1 cup chopped carrots
½ medium yellow bell pepper, stemmed, seeded, and chopped
1 teaspoon dried oregano
1 teaspoon dried thyme
1 teaspoon dried basil
¼ teaspoon salt
¼ teaspoon freshly ground black pepper
2 tablespoons extra-virgin olive oil
1 tablespoon unsalted butter

1. Place all ingredients in a large, uncovered pot with 2 cups of hot water and bring to a boil. Reduce heat and cook on low heat for 40 to 45 minutes. Occasionally taste for richness of flavor and correct seasonings.

SIDES

ORANGE AND FENNEL SLAW

HERB-CRUSTED BEEFSTEAK TOMATOES

BARLEY WITH GRAPEFRUIT, SPINACH, AND ALMONDS

QUINOA–WHITE BEAN CAKES

GINGER-GLAZED CARROTS

ITALIAN STEWED GREEN BEANS

SPINACH FUSILLI WITH ROASTED MUSHROOMS

MUSTARD-CHILI WHIPPED SWEET POTATOES

WHITE BEAN AND CARROT SMASH

SPICY TOMATO STEWED CAULIFLOWER

ORANGE AND FENNEL SLAW

SERVES 4

Nutritional Information Per Serving: 61 cal., 0 g fat, 0 g sat. fat, 14 g carb., 2 g protein, 288 mg sodium, 3 g sugar, 4 g fiber.

2 bulbs fennel, trimmed and fronds reserved
1 large navel orange
2 tablespoons rice vinegar
½ teaspoon Dijon mustard
¼ teaspoon salt
4 scallions, thinly sliced

1. Halve the fennel vertically through the core. Cut the woody core away from the bulbs. Using a mandolin slicer or a sharp knife, slice the fennel bulb halves crosswise into paper-thin slices and transfer them to a medium bowl.

2. Stand the orange upright and, with a sharp knife, cut away the peel and white pith and discard. Hold the orange in one hand, and using the knife, carefully cut the segments away from the membrane into a bowl. Coarsely chop the orange segments and add them to the fennel; squeeze the membrane into the empty bowl to remove as much juice as possible and discard the membrane. Add the rice vinegar, Dijon, and salt to the orange juice and whisk well to combine. Drizzle the dressing over the fennel and toss well to coat.

3. Coarsely chop the reserve fennel fronds and add them to the slaw along with the scallions. Toss well until combined; refrigerate until ready to serve.

HERB-CRUSTED BEEFSTEAK TOMATOES

SERVES 4

Nutritional Information Per Serving: 101 cal., 7 g fat, 1 g sat. fat, 8 g carb., 1 g protein, 232 mg sodium, 2 g sugar, 1 g fiber

Cooking spray
2 large beefsteak tomatoes (about 1 pound), halved horizontally
½ cup panko bread crumbs
2 tablespoons extra-virgin olive oil
1 tablespoon chopped fresh parsley
1 teaspoon chopped fresh sage
1 teaspoon chopped fresh thyme leaves
¼ teaspoon salt
¼ teaspoon freshly ground black pepper

1. Preheat the oven to 350 degrees F.

2. Spray a shallow baking dish with cooking spray and set the tomato halves cut-side-up in the dish.

3. In a small bowl, stir the bread crumbs, oil, parsley, sage, thyme, salt, and pepper together until combined. Sprinkle one-fourth of the mixture evenly over the top of each tomato. Roast in the oven until the tomato is very soft and the bread crumbs are golden, 20 to 25 minutes.

4. Serve warm.

BARLEY WITH GRAPEFRUIT, SPINACH, AND ALMONDS

SERVES 4

2 cups rinsed and cooked pearl barley

¾ ruby grapefruit

1 tablespoon whole-grain mustard

½ teaspoon honey

2 tablespoons extra-virgin olive oil

¼ teaspoon salt

¼ teaspoon freshly ground black pepper

4 cups baby spinach leaves

⅓ cup sliced almonds, toasted

Nutritional Information Per Serving: 345 cal., 12 g fat, 1 g sat. fat, 26 g carb., 7 g protein, 261 mg sodium, 17 g sugar, 8 g fiber

1. Put the barley in a medium bowl. Set the grapefruit on a work surface and, using a sharp knife, cut the peel and white membrane away from fruit, exposing the segments. Hold the grapefruit in one hand and, using the knife, cut the segments away from the membrane and drop them on the work surface. Halve the grapefruit segments crosswise and add them to the barley.

2. Squeeze the grapefruit membrane over a small bowl, removing as much juice as possible. Add the mustard, honey, oil, salt, and pepper to the grapefruit juice and whisk well until combined and thickened. Add the spinach and almonds to the barley and toss well to combine. Drizzle the dressing over the salad and stir until well coated.

3. Serve at room temperature or chilled.

QUINOA–WHITE BEAN CAKES

SERVES 4

Nutritional Information Per Serving: 194 cal., 2 g fat, 1 g sat. fat, 30 g carb., 10 g protein, 210 mg sodium, 5 g sugar, 8 g fiber

1 can (15-ounce) low-sodium white beans, drained
1 cup cooked quinoa
1 large egg
1 teaspoon Dijon mustard
1 teaspoon dried basil
½ teaspoon garlic powder
¼ teaspoon salt
¼ teaspoon freshly ground black pepper
½ cup panko bread crumbs
Cooking spray

1. Preheat the oven to 375° F.

2. Line a baking sheet with parchment paper.

3. Put the beans in a medium bowl and mash two-thirds of them with a potato masher. Add the quinoa and mix with the beans until evenly combined. In another small bowl, whisk the egg, mustard, basil, garlic powder, salt, and pepper together until combined and pour it over the bean mixture. Stir the mixture with a wooden spoon until evenly mixed.

4. Put the bread crumbs on a plate. Using wet hands, divide the mixture into 8 portions and fold them into small, flat cakes about ½-inch thick. Roll the cakes in the bread crumbs, pressing on the cakes to cause the bread crumbs to adhere. Transfer the breaded

cakes to the baking sheet and spray them lightly with cooking spray. Bake in the oven until the cakes turn light golden and are set, 12 to 15 minutes.

5. Serve warm.

GINGER-GLAZED CARROTS

SERVES 4

1 pound carrots, peeled and sliced
   ¼-inch thick
¼ cup orange juice
2 teaspoons fresh ginger, peeled and
   finely grated
1 tablespoon unsalted butter
¼ teaspoon salt

Nutritional Information Per Serving: 70 cal., 3 g fat, 2 g sat. fat, 14 g carb., 0 g protein, 256 mg sodium, 5 g sugar, 4 g fiber

1. Fill a large saucepan with water and bring to a boil over medium-high heat. Add the carrots and cook until just tender, 8 to 10 minutes and drain.

2. Meanwhile, bring the orange juice to a simmer over medium-low heat. Stir in the ginger and cook until the juice has reduced and thickened, about 5 minutes. Stir in the butter, add the carrots and stir gently until very hot and glazed.

3. Serve warm.

ITALIAN STEWED GREEN BEANS

SERVES 4

1 tablespoon extra-virgin olive oil
1 medium yellow onion, sliced
2 cloves garlic, chopped
1 can (15-ounce) no-salt-added Italian stewed tomatoes
1 tablespoon balsamic vinegar
Pinch red pepper flakes
One pound fresh green beans, trimmed
¼ teaspoon salt

Nutritional Information Per Serving: 113 cal., 4 g fat, 1 g sat. fat, 19 g carb., 5 g protein, 183 mg sodium, 7 g sugar, 5 g fiber

1. Heat the oil in a large skillet over medium heat. Add the onion and cook, stirring occasionally, until softened, about 5 minutes. Add the garlic and tomatoes and bring the mixture to a simmer. Cover and cook for 5 minutes.

2. Stir in the vinegar, pepper flakes, beans, and salt. Cover and cook until the beans are crisp-tender, 6 to 8 minutes.

3. Serve warm.

SPINACH FUSILLI WITH ROASTED MUSHROOMS

SERVES 4

4 ounces sliced button mushrooms

2 shallots, chopped

2 tablespoons extra-virgin olive oil

1½ cups low-sodium vegetable broth

8 ounces spinach fusilli

1 tablespoon unsalted butter

¼ teaspoon salt

¼ teaspoon freshly ground black pepper

¼ cup finely grated parmesan cheese

Nutritional Information Per Serving: 341 cal., 13 g fat, 4 g sat. fat, 38 g carb., 15 g protein, 317 mg sodium, 5 g sugar, 4 g fiber

1. Preheat the oven to 375° F.

2. Put the mushrooms and shallots on a nonstick baking sheet. Drizzle the oil over them and toss to coat. Roast in the oven, stirring several times, until the mushrooms and shallots begin to brown, 12 to 15 minutes. Remove from the oven.

3. Meanwhile, bring a large pot of water to a boil over medium-high heat.

4. Pour the vegetable broth into a large skillet and bring it to a simmer over medium heat. Cook until reduced to about ½ cup, 6 to 8 minutes. Drop the pasta into the boiling water and cook according to the package instructions then drain.

5. Whisk the butter into the reduced vegetable broth. Add the pasta and mushroom mixture and stir to coat evenly. Season with the salt and pepper, remove the pan from the heat and stir in the parmesan cheese.

6. Serve warm.

MUSTARD-CHILI WHIPPED SWEET POTATOES

SERVES 4

Nutritional Information Per Serving: 138 cal., 1 g fat, 0 g sat. fat, 32 g carb., 5 g protein, 335 mg sodium, 11 g sugar, 6 g fiber

1¼ pounds sweet potatoes, peeled and chopped

¼ nonfat Greek yogurt

1 tablespoon whole-grain Dijon mustard

½ teaspoon salt

½ teaspoon chili powder

¼ teaspoon freshly ground black pepper

1. Put the potatoes in a medium saucepan and cover with water. Bring the potatoes to a boil over medium-high heat and cook until they are fork-tender, about 10 minutes. Drain the potatoes and transfer them to a mixing bowl or stand mixer.

2. Add the yogurt, mustard, salt, chili powder, and pepper to the potatoes and whip with a hand-held mixer or stand mixer with the paddle attachment until completely smooth. Serve warm.

WHITE BEAN AND CARROT SMASH

SERVES 4

Nutritional Information Per Serving: 105 cal., 0 g fat, 0 g sat. fat, 19 g carb., 7 g protein, 336 mg sodium, 2 g sugar, 7 g fiber

2 medium carrots, peeled and chopped

1 large garlic clove, smashed

1 small bay leaf

1 can (14-ounce) low-sodium white beans, drained and rinsed

1 teaspoon Dijon mustard

¼ teaspoon salt

1. Put the carrots, garlic, and bay leaf into a medium saucepan and cover with water. Bring the mixture to a boil over medium-high heat. Cover and cook until the carrots are very soft and fork-tender, about 20 minutes.

2. When the carrots are cooked, add the beans to the pan and cook for several minutes until they are hot. Drain the vegetables and discard the bay leaf. Return the vegetables to the pan and, using a potato masher, coarsely mash the carrots, being sure to mash up the garlic completely. Add the mustard and salt and mix well until combined. Serve warm.

SPICY TOMATO STEWED CAULIFLOWER

SERVES 4

Nutritional Information Per Serving: 71 cal., 0 g fat, 0 g sat. fat, 17 g carb., 2 g protein, 216 mg sodium, 11 g sugar, 3 g fiber

1 can (14-ounce) Italian-flavored stewed tomatoes
½ cup water
1 small red onion, sliced
½ teaspoon red chili flakes
Pinch chili powder
2 cups small cauliflower florets (from about ½ head)

1. Put the tomatoes, water, onion, chili flakes, and chili powder into a medium sauce pan and bring to a boil over medium-high heat. Cook for about 5 minutes until the liquid evaporates slightly.

2. Add the cauliflower, reduce the heat to medium low, cover, and simmer, stirring very frequently, until the cauliflower is soft when pierced with a knife but not mushy, 6 to 8 minutes.

3. Serve warm.

SMOOTHIES

These smoothies are low in calories, low in carbohydrates, and full of vitamins, minerals, and other important phytonutrients. They are easy to make and extremely filling. Pay attention to the number of servings that the recipe yields and only eat one serving at a particular meal. If you need to substitute ingredients, make sure you keep in mind the amount of carbohydrates and calories that the substitution could be adding to the recipe.

THE ENERGIZER

ORANGE PARADISO

BLUEBERRY TWISTER

THE MOLTEN RAZZY

PURPLE PANACHE

THE POPEYE

CHILLY COCONUT

THE HONEY BUZZ

THE BLUEBERRY MASH

ANTIOXIDANT SUPREME

THE ENERGIZER

SERVES 2
SERVING SIZE: 12 OUNCES

1 cup peeled, seeded, and chopped papaya

½ cup frozen pineapple chunks

½ cup frozen peach slices

½ cup low-fat kefir

½ cup unsweetened coconut milk

Juice of ½ lime

1 tablespoon unfiltered organic flaxseed oil

½ tablespoon raw organic honey

Nutritional Information Per Serving: 270 cal., 18 g fat, 10 g sat. fat, 28 g carb., 4 g protein, 59 mg sodium, 16 g sugar, 3 g fiber

1. Combine all ingredients in a blender and purée until smooth. Enjoy!

ORANGE PARADISO

SERVES 2
SERVING SIZE: 12 OUNCES

½ cup frozen blueberries

½ cup frozen raspberries

½ cup frozen strawberry slices

½ cup tightly packed Swiss chard, stems and ribs removed

½ cup fresh orange juice

Juice of 1 large juice, navel, or Valencia orange

1 tablespoon unfiltered flaxseed oil

10 ice cubes

Nutritional Information Per Serving: 139 cal., 7 g fat, 1 g sat. fat, 19 g carb., 2 g protein, 20 mg sodium, 12 g sugar, 3 g fiber

1. Combine all ingredients in a blender and purée until smooth. Enjoy!

BLUEBERRY TWISTER

SERVES 2
SERVING SIZE: 12 OUNCES

1 cup fresh blueberries (substitute frozen blueberries out of season)

1 cup chilled coconut water (substitute cold-pressed apple juice if you prefer a sweeter drink)

½ cup loosely packed baby spinach, stems removed

1 ripe small banana, peeled and sliced

Juice of 1 small lemon

2 tablespoons unfiltered flaxseed oil

10 ice cubes

Nutritional Information Per Serving: 238 cal., 14 g fat, 2 g sat. fat, 30 g carb., 2 g protein, 67 mg sodium, 19 g sugar, 4 g fiber

1. Combine all ingredients in a blender and purée until smooth. Enjoy!

THE MOLTEN RAZZY

SERVES 2
SERVING SIZE: 12 OUNCES

Nutritional Information Per Serving: 322 cal., 27 g fat, 19 g sat. fat, 24 g carb., 3 g protein, 59 mg sodium, 17 g sugar, 7 g fiber

1 cup frozen raspberries
¾ cup unsweetened coconut milk
1 ripe small banana
¼ cup water
1 tablespoon raspberry yogurt
½ tablespoon semisweet dark chocolate baking chips
1 teaspoon unfiltered flaxseed oil
1 teaspoon ground chia seeds
1½ teaspoons organic chocolate hemp protein powder (substitute organic chocolate whey protein powder)
10 ice cubes

1. Combine all ingredients in a blender and purée until smooth. Enjoy!

PURPLE PANACHE

SERVES: 2
SERVING SIZE: 12 OUNCES

¾ cup frozen blueberries
1 cup loosely packed baby spinach, stems removed
¾ cup almond milk
1 ripe small banana, sliced
¼ cup low-fat plain yogurt
½ cup sliced fresh strawberries
½ teaspoon fresh ginger, peeled and grated

Nutritional Information Per Serving: 166 cal., 3 g fat, 1 g sat. fat, 22 g carb., 6 g protein, 131 mg sodium, 10 g sugar, 5 g fiber

1. Combine all ingredients in a blender and purée until smooth. Enjoy!

THE POPEYE

SERVES: 2
SERVING SIZE: 12 OUNCES

1 small banana, sliced
¾ cup loosely packed baby spinach
¼ cup low-fat plain yogurt
½ cup freshly squeezed orange juice
½ small lemon, peeled and seeded
½ lime, peeled and seeded
1 tablespoon unfiltered organic flaxseed oil
8 ice cubes

Nutritional Information Per Serving: 248 cal., 15 g fat, 2 g sat. fat, 18 g carb., 5 g protein, 56 mg sodium, 9 g sugar, 2 g fiber

1. Combine all ingredients in a blender and purée until smooth. Enjoy!

CHILLY COCONUT

SERVES 2
SERVING SIZE: 12 OUNCES

¾ cup frozen pineapple chunks
1 small ripe banana, peeled and sliced
¼ cup shredded unsweetened coconut
½ cup coconut water

Nutritional Information Per Serving: 158 cal., 7 g fat, 6 g sat. fat, 25 g carb., 3 g protein, 67 mg sodium, 10 g sugar, 4 g fiber

1. Combine all ingredients in a blender and purée until smooth. Enjoy!

THE HONEY BUZZ

SERVES 2
SERVING SIZE: 12 OUNCES

½ cup frozen strawberries
½ cup sliced Honeycrisp apples
½ small ripe banana
½ cup low-fat milk (or substitute soy milk)
1 tablespoon bee pollen
4 ice cubes

Nutritional Information Per Serving: 84 cal., 1 g fat, 0 g sat. fat, 19 g carb., 2 g protein, 23 mg sodium, 11 g sugar, 3 g fiber

1. Combine all ingredients in a blender and purée until smooth. Enjoy!

THE BLUEBERRY MASH

SERVES 2
SERVING SIZE: 12 OUNCES

½ small ripe banana, peeled and sliced
½ cup frozen blueberries
¼ cup low-fat plain yogurt
½ cup low-fat milk (or substitute soy or almond milk)
½ teaspoon unfiltered organic flaxseed oil

Nutritional Information Per Serving: 116 cal., 3 g fat, 1 g sat. fat, 18 g carb., 6 g protein, 70 mg sodium, 10 g sugar, 3 g fiber

1. Combine all ingredients in a blender and purée until smooth. Enjoy!

ANTIOXIDANT SUPREME

SERVES 2
SERVING SIZE: 12 OUNCES

½ cup frozen blueberries
½ cup frozen cherries
½ cup frozen strawberries
½ small ripe banana, peeled and sliced
½ cup orange juice (not from concentrate)
4 ice cubes

Nutritional Information Per Serving: 103 cal., 0 g fat, 0 g sat. fat, 25 g carb., 2 g protein, 0 mg sodium, 18 g sugar, 3 g fiber

1. Combine all ingredients in a blender and purée until smooth. Enjoy!

EPILOGUE

Sugar is one of the most addictive food ingredients on earth. It causes chemical changes in our brain that signal pleasure and prompt our reward system to want more and more. All sugar is not "bad," but too much sugar and some forms of sugar are unhealthy and part of the cause for many illnesses. Reducing the amount of sugar you consume and making strategic choices about where you get this sugar can be critical to good health.

Blasting sugar out of your diet is not easy, but it can be done. As with anything else that is addictive, breaking the cycle will take some adjustments. You will literally feel the sugar leaving your body and this might manifest in the form of headaches, mood swings, erratic energy swings, and a general feeling of unease. But don't worry, as this is a sign that your body is purging and freeing the grip that sugar has held for far too long.

Living a life without sugar in some form is almost impossible, but dramatically reducing added sugars is very realistic and sustainable. With this plan, you should be well on your way to a life of eating and feeling better. It's still okay to indulge in an occasional slice of cake or a piece of candy, as consuming these foods in moderation will not do any real harm. But you will now find that you don't have to over-indulge in these sweets, as an occasional treat is enough to satisfy your craving. If you find yourself losing your way, go right back to week 1 of this program and do as much as you need to get back in the groove. Food should be fun, but it also should be nourishing. You now have the tools. So eat well and live well and never be afraid to Blast the Sugar Out!

APPENDIX 1

SUGAR SWAPS

Below you will find some sugar swaps that can reduce your carbohydrate and sugar load. Feel free to make other swaps that are not listed. Choosing whole grains over refined grains is almost always the better choice.

Snickers *SWITCH* Slice of toast spread with a tablespoon of Nutella

White bread *SWITCH* Ezekiel

Soda *SWITCH* Iced tea (with a little stevia if you want to sweeten it)

Frosted cereal *SWITCH* Oatmeal

Bottled salad dressing *SWITCH* Olive oil

Yogurt with added fruit *SWITCH* Greek yogurt (add your own fruit)

Sodas or fruit juice *SWITCH* Water/unsweetened tea

Whole milk *SWITCH* Skim or reduced-fat milk

Full-fat cheese *SWITCH* Reduced-fat cheese

Plain bagel with cream cheese *SWITCH* Whole-grain bagel or English muffin topped with organic peanut butter with no added sugar

White rice *SWITCH* Brown rice or quinoa

White pasta *SWITCH* Whole-wheat or whole-grain pasta

Fruit juice (non-squeezed) *SWITCH* Whole fruit

Granola bar *SWITCH* Cacao nibs + almonds

Chips or pretzels *SWITCH* Raw veggies or fruit

White baked potatoes *SWITCH* Sweet baked potatoes or yams

Spaghetti *SWITCH* Spaghetti squash

Regular pizza crust *SWITCH* Thin pizza crust

Cashews *SWITCH* Walnuts

Cake frosting *SWITCH* Dusting of powdered sugar

12-inch flour tortilla *SWITCH* 6-inch flour tortilla

Dried fruit (e.g., plums, bananas, mango) *SWITCH* Fresh sliced fruit

Breaded chicken *SWITCH* Grilled chicken

Macaroni salad *SWITCH* Spinach and vinegar salad

Granola *SWITCH* Oatmeal

White flour *SWITCH* Whole-wheat flour

White granulated sugar *SWITCH* Applesauce

Frosting *SWITCH* Marshmallow fluff

Cream *SWITCH* Evaporated skim milk

White rice *SWITCH* Steamed cauliflower

Mashed potatoes *SWITCH* Mashed cauliflower

Bread crumbs *SWITCH* Old-fashioned rolled oats

2 slices of whole-wheat bread *SWITCH* 4-inch whole-wheat pita

Tortilla wraps *SWITCH* Lettuce leaves

Instant oatmeal *SWITCH* Steel-cut oatmeal

Honey-roasted peanuts *SWITCH* Dry-roasted peanuts

Ice cream sundae *SWITCH* Yogurt parfait made with nonfat vanilla yogurt and fresh berries

Smoothie with a base of fruit juice *SWITCH* Smoothie with a base of almond milk

Milk chocolate *SWITCH* 70 percent Dark chocolate

White cream sauce *SWITCH* Marinara sauce

Jams and jellies *SWITCH* All-fruit spreads

Ketchup *SWITCH* Salsa, sliced tomatoes, or sun-dried tomato hummus

Pancakes made with white flour *SWITCH* Whole-grain pancakes

Waffles made with white flour *SWITCH* Whole-grain waffles

Boxed cereal *SWITCH* Steel-cut oatmeal

Fried egg, bacon, American cheese, English muffin *SWITCH* Scrambled egg whites, onion, tomato, spinach, whole-grain tortilla

Ice cream sundaes *SWITCH* Parfait using low-fat vanilla yogurt, fresh berries, and 1 tablespoon of granola

Popsicle *SWITCH* Frozen grapes

Honey-roasted peanuts *SWITCH* Dry-roasted peanuts

French fries *SWITCH* Baked sweet potato fries

Margarita *SWITCH* Red wine

Ice cream *SWITCH* Puréed frozen bananas + almonds

Pizza *SWITCH* Whole-wheat pita with no-sugar-added tomato sauce and shredded part-skim mozzarella

Hamburger *SWITCH* Portobello mushroom

Mayonnaise *SWITCH* Avocado spread

Creamy salad dressing *SWITCH* Olive oil and balsamic vinegar with a pinch of salt and pepper to taste

Iceberg lettuce *SWITCH* Raw spinach

Sour cream *SWITCH* Greek yogurt

Sugar *SWITCH* Cinnamon

APPENDIX 2

CARDIOVASCULAR/AEROBIC EXERCISES

Below is a list of exercises that you can do to complete the exercise portion of the program. This list is only suggestive and is not meant to be complete. Rather than perform the exercises at the same pace for a prolonged period of time, try to train in intervals. Interval training means that you alternate periods of high exertion with periods of low exertion or rest. For example, if you're riding a bicycle, sprint as hard as you can for 30 seconds, then pedal slowly for 30 seconds. After this slow-pedaling period, go hard again for 30 seconds, then slow for the next 30. Do as much as you can for up to 15 minutes, then try another exercise such as high knees. Do the same type of intervals with this exercise. This type of training is called *high intensity interval training* (HIIT) and has been shown to be more effective at burning calories, increasing metabolism, and accelerating weight loss. For a more specific description of these exercises go to www.shredlife.com.

Bicycle

Burpees (Squat Thrusts)
1. Stand with your feet spread hip-width apart and your arms resting down by your side. Put more of your weight on the front portion of your feet with your heels slightly off the ground.

2. Lower yourself into a squat position, making sure you steady yourself by placing your hands flat on the floor in front of you.

3. Once you reach the squat position and your hands are on the floor, quickly kick your legs backward so that your body is extended into a push-up position.

4. Lower your chest to an inch above the floor, just as you would if doing a push-up. Make sure you don't let your chest hit the floor.

5. In one motion, push your chest back up and kick your legs forward so that you're back into a squat position.

6. From the squat position, use your legs to push off the ground and jump as high as you can into the air, then repeat from step 1 again.

Dancing

Elliptical machine

High knees

1. Stand straight with your feet apart no wider than your hips. Make sure your arms are hanging down by your side and your back is straight as you look forward.

2. Jump from one foot to another as if running in place, making sure that you lift your knees as high as possible.

3. Your arms should be bent to ninety degrees with your hands clamped into a fist. Pump your arms up and down in the same motion as your legs.

4. Be light on your feet, so make sure your heels never strike the ground, but only the balls of your feet as you continue the jumping motion for the duration of the exercise. Touch the ground with the balls of your feet, as lightly as possible, and continuing jumping.

Ice skaters

Think about the motion of competitive speed skaters as they move around the rink.

1. Start with your feet a little wider than your shoulders. Looking directly forward, keep your back straight and your knees slightly bent.

2. In one motion, take your right leg and extend it behind you toward the left side of your body so that it is further left than your left leg. Take your left hand and bend down toward the right side of your body and touch the ground.

3. Next, do the same motion, but switch sides. Bring your right leg back to its starting position and at the same time bring your left leg across behind the right side of your body. At the same time touch the ground in front of your left side with your right hand.

4. Repeat this alternating movement for the desired number of reps.

Jumping rope

Mountain climbers

1. Starting Position: Start as if in a push-up position with your hands, however, wider than your shoulders and in front. Slightly elevate your buttocks, but not too high. Start with your left foot forward until it comes to rest on the floor under your chest. At this point your left knee and hip are bent, and your thigh is in toward your chest. Your right knee should be off the ground, making your right leg extended straight and strong. Your right toes are tucked under, heel up. Contract your abdominal muscles to stabilize your spine.

2. Keep your hands firmly on the ground and jump, so that you can switch leg positions. Now your left leg is extended straight behind you and your right leg is bent underneath your chest with your right foot on the floor. Be sure to keep your abdominals engaged and shoulders strong. Do not lift your buttocks too high, as that will defeat the purpose of the exercise. Keep your head up and looking forward.

Exercise Variation: If you have a physical impairment that limits the range of motion in your hips, place your hands on a step or platform for better leverage.

Don't shift all of your weight forward onto your front foot. Your weight should remain evenly distributed on both legs. Do not shift all your weight forward into your front foot.

Rowing

Running

Skating

Soccer

Stairmaster

Swimming

Tennis

Treadmill

Walking

Walking up and down stairs

INDEX